BELIEVE IT OR NOT. . . .

- One cigarette can destroy up to 100 mg. of vitamin C!
- Lecithin can provide the same stick-free pots and pans that Pam does—without propellents!
- Milk with synthetic vitamin D can rob the body of magnesium!
- People who live in smoggy cities are not getting the vitamin D that their country cousins get because the smog absorbs the sun's ultraviolet rays!
- More than one cocktail a day can cause a depletion of vitamins B_1, B_6 and folic acid!
- Oral contraceptives (The Pill) can interfere with the availability of vitamins B_6, B_{12}, folic acid and vitamin C!
- Cancer researchers at the Massachusetts Institute of Technology have found that vitamins C and E and certain chemicals called indoles, found in cabbage, Brussels sprouts, and related vegetables in the crucifer family, are potent and safe inhibitors of certain carcinogens!
- Vitamins B_1 and B_6 can help fight air- and seasickness!
- If you're on a high-protein $diet$ ⋯⋯⋯⋯ or B_6 *increases*!

It's all l⋯⋯

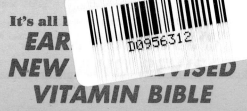

EAR⋯
NEW ⋯⋯⋯ⅤISED
VITAMIN BIBLE

Also by Earl Mindell

**Earl Mindell's Shaping Up With Vitamins
Unsafe At Any Meal**

Published by
WARNER BOOKS

Earl Mindell's
NEW AND REVISED

Vitamin Bible

How the Right Vitamins and Nutrient Supplements
Can Help Turn Your Life Around

Earl Mindell

WARNER BOOKS

A Warner Communications Company

WARNER BOOKS EDITION

This Warner Books Edition is published by arrangement
with Rawson Associates, 597 Fifth Avenue, New York,
N.Y. 10017

Warner Books, Inc.
666 Fifth Avenue
New York, N.Y. 10103

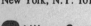 A Warner Communications Company

Printed in the United States of America

First Warner Books Printing: May, 1985

Reissued: September, 1988

20   19   18

This book is dedicated to
GAIL, ALANNA, EVAN,
our parents and families
and to
the future

The first wealth is health.

RALPH WALDO EMERSON
"The Conduct of Life"

Acknowledgments

I wish to express my deep and lasting appreciation to my friends and associates who have assisted me in the preparation of this book, especially J. Kenney, Ph.D.; Linus Pauling, Ph.D.; Harold Segal, Ph.D.; Bernard Bubman, R.Ph.; Mel Rich, R.Ph.; Sal Messinero, R.Ph.; Arnold Fox, M.D.; Dennis Huddleson, M.D.; Stuart Fisher, M.D.; Robert Mendelson, M.D.; Gershon Lesser, M.D.; David Velkoff, M.D.; Rory Jaffee, M.D.; Vickie Hufnagel, M.D,.; Donald Cruden, O.D.; Joel Strom, D.D.S.; Nathan Sperling, D.D.S.; Peter Mallory; and Hester Mundis.

I would also like to thank the Nutrition Foundation; the International College of Applied Nutrition; the American Medical Association; the New York Blood Center; the American Academy of Pediatrics; the American Dietetic Association; the National Academy of Sciences; the National Dairy Council; the Society for Nutrition Education; the United Fresh Fruit and Vegetable Association; the Albany College of Pharmacy; Edward Leavitt, D.V.M.; Jane Bix, D.V.M.; Betty Haskins; Stephanie Marco; Susan Towison; Ronald Borenstein; Laura Borenstein; and Richard Curtis, without whom a project of this scope could never have been completed.

Contents

A Note to the Reader About This Newly Revised Edition

Since the first publication of *The Vitamin Bible* in 1979, the field of vitamins and nutrition has exploded. More people than ever before in history are taking supplements, and startling new discoveries about the interrelation between vitamins, drugs, natural foods, and health are being made daily. Preventative medicine is no longer a fad, but a fact—as attested to by the conservative National Academy of Sciences' recent report that 80–85 percent of all human internal cancers could be prevented through improved nutrition.

Other new discoveries, such as how the right foods and supplements can effectively substitute for drugs, alleviate the discomforts of premenstrual syndrome (PMS), rejuvenate the metabolism, improve the immune system, reduce the risk of heart disease, act as natural painkillers, fatigue reducers, and much more, are included in this new expanded edition, along with complete new sections on amino acids, herbs, and the latest cautions about them all.

ONE IMPORTANT REMINDER

The regimens throughout this book are recommendations, not prescriptions, and are not intended as medical advice. Before starting any new program, check with your physician or a nutritionally oriented doctor (see section 278), especially if you have a specific physical problem or are taking any medication.

Preface

This book is written for *you*—the untold legions of men and women who are forever trying to fit yourselves into statistical norms only to find that the charts are designed for some mythical average person who is taller, shorter, fatter, skinnier, less or more active than you'll ever be. It is a guide to healthy living for individuals, not statistics. Wherever feasible I have given personal advice, for this, I believe, is the only way to lead anyone to optimal health, which is the purpose of this book.

In these pages I have combined my knowledge of pharmacy with that of nutrition to best explain the confusing, often dangerous, interrelation of drugs and vitamins. I've attempted to personalize and be specific so as to eliminate much of the confusion about vitamins that has arisen with generalizations.

In using the book you will occasionally find that your vitamin needs fall into several different categories. In this case, let common sense dictate the necessary adjustment. (If you are already taking B_6, for example, there's no need to double up on it unless a higher dosage is called for.)

The recommendations I've made are not meant to be prescriptive but can easily be used as flexible programs when working with your doctor. No book can substitute for professional care.

It is my sincerest hope that I have provided you with information that will help you attain the longest, happiest, and healthiest of lives.

EARL MINDELL, R.Ph., Ph.D.

I

Getting into Vitamins

1. Why I Did

My professional education was strictly establishment when it came to vitamins. My courses in pharmacology, biochemistry, organic and inorganic chemistry, and public health hardly dealt with vitamins at all—except in relation to deficiency diseases. Lack of vitamin C? Scurvy. Out of B_1? Beriberi. Not enough vitamin D? Rickets. My courses were the standard fare, with the usual references to a balanced diet and eating the "right foods" (all unappetizingly illustrated on semiglossy charts).

There were no references to vitamins being used for disease prevention or as ways to optimum health.

> Both of us were working fifteen hours a day,
> but only *I* looked and felt it.

In 1965 I opened my first pharmacy. Until then I never realized just how many drugs people were taking, not for illness but simply to get through the day. (I had one regular patron who had prescriptions for pills to supplant virtually all his bodily functions—and he wasn't even sick!) My partner at the time was very vitamin-oriented. Both of us were working fifteen hours a day, but only *I* looked and felt it. When I asked him what his secret was, he said it was no secret at all. It was vitamins. I realized what he was talking about had very little to do with scurvy and beriberi and a lot to do with me. I instantly became an eager pupil and have never since regretted it. He taught me the benefits that could be reaped from nature's own foods in the form of vitamins, how B complex and C could alleviate stress, how vitamin E would increase my endurance and stamina, and how B_{12} could eliminate fatigue. After embarking on the most elementary vitamin regimens I was not only convinced. I was converted.

Suddenly nutrition became the most important thing in my life. I read every book I could find on the subject, clipped articles and tracked down their sources, dug out my pharmacy school texts and discovered the amazingly close relationship that did indeed exist between biochemistry and nutrition. I attended any health lecture I could. In fact, it was at one such lecture that I learned of the RNA-DNA nucleic complex and its age-reversing properties. (I have been taking RNA-DNA supplements since then, as well as SOD—Super-Oxide Dismutase—and DHEA—Dehydroepiandrosterone—a natural anti-obesity and antiaging agent. Today, because of these, most people guess me to be five to ten years younger than I am.) I was excited about each new discovery in the field, and it showed.

A whole new world had opened up for me and I wanted others to share it. My partner understood completely. We began giving out samples of B complex and B_{12} tablets to patrons, suggesting they try decreasing their dependency on tranquilizers, pep pills, and sedatives with the vitamins and vitamin-rich foods.

The results were remarkable! People kept coming back to tell us how much better and more energetic they felt. Instead of the negativity and resignation that often accompanies drug therapies, we received overwhelming positiveness. I saw a woman who had spent nearly all her young adult life on Librium, running from doctor to therapist and back again, become a healthy, happy, drug-free human being; a sixty-year-old architect, on the brink of retirement because of ill health, regain his well-being and accept a commission for what is now one of the foremost office buildings in Los Angeles; a middle-aged pill-dependent actor kick his habit and land a sought-after supporting role in a TV series that still nets him handsome residuals.

By 1970 I was totally committed to nutrition and preventive medicine. Seeing the paucity of knowledge in the area, I went into partnership with another pharmacist for the prime purpose of making natural vitamins and accurate nutrition information available to the public.

Today, as a nutritionist, lecturer, and author, I'm still excited about that world that opened up to me over twenty years ago—a world that continues to grow with new discoveries daily—and I'm eager to share it.

2. What Vitamins Are

> We must obtain vitamins from natural foods
> or dietary supplements in order
> to sustain life.

When I mention the word "vitamin," most people think "pill." Thinking "pill" brings to mind confusing images of medicine and drugs. Though vitamins can and certainly often do do the work of both medicine and drugs, they are neither.

• Quite simply, vitamins are organic substances necessary for life. Vitamins are essential to the normal functioning of our bodies and, save for a few exceptions, cannot be manufactured or synthesized internally. Necessary for our growth, vitality, and general well-being, they are found in minute quantities in all natural food. We must obtain vitamins from these foods or from dietary supplements.

What you have to keep in mind is that supplements, which are available in tablet, capsule, liquid, powder, and even injection forms, are still just food substances and, unless synthetic, are also derived from living plants and animals.

• It is impossible to sustain life without *all* the essential vitamins.

3. What Vitamins Are Not

Vitamins are neither pep pills nor
substitutes for food.

A lot of people think vitamins can replace food. They cannot. In fact, vitamins cannot be assimilated without ingesting food. There are a lot of erroneous beliefs about vitamins, and I hope this book can clear up most of them.

• Vitamins are not pep pills and have no caloric or energy value of their own.
• Vitamins are not substitutes for protein or for any

other nutrients, such as minerals, fats, carbohydrates, water—or even for each other!
• Vitamins themselves are not the components of our body structures.
• You cannot take vitamins, stop eating, and expect to be healthy.

4. How They Work

If you think of the body as an automobile's combustion engine and vitamins as spark plugs, you have a fairly good idea of how these amazing minute food substances work for us.

Vitamins regulate our metabolism through enzyme systems. A single deficiency can endanger the whole body.

Vitamins are components of our enzyme systems which, acting like spark plugs, energize and regulate our metabolism, keeping us tuned up and functioning at high performance.

Compared with our intake of other nutrients like proteins, fats, and carbohydrates, our vitamin intake (even on some megadose regimens) is minuscule. But a deficiency in even one vitamin can endanger the whole human body.

5. Should You Take Supplements?

"Everyone who has in the past eaten sugar, white flour, or canned food has some deficiency disease. . . ."

Since vitamins occur in all organic material, some containing more of one vitamin than another and in greater or lesser amounts, you could say that if you ate the "right" foods in a well-balanced diet, you would get all the vitamins you need. And you would probably be right. The problem is, very few of us are able to arrange this mythical diet. According to Dr. Daniel T. Quigley, author of *The National Malnutrition,* "Everyone who has in the past eaten processed sugar, white flour, or canned food has some deficiency disease, the extent of the disease depending on the percentage of such deficient food in the diet."

Because most restaurants tend to reheat food or keep it warm under heat lamps, if you frequently eat out, you run the risk of vitamin A, B₁, and C deficiencies. (And if you're a woman between the ages of thirteen and forty, this sort of work-saving dining is likely to cost you invaluable calcium and iron.)

Most of the foods we eat have been processed and depleted in nutrients. Take breads and cereals, for example. Practically all of them you find in today's supermarkets are high in nothing but carbohydrates. "But they are enriched!" you say. It's written right on the label: *Enriched.*

Enriched? The standard of enrichment for white flour is to replace the twenty-two natural nutrients that are removed with three B vitamins, vitamin D, calcium, and iron salts. Now really, for the staff of life, that seems a pretty flimsy stick.

I think you can see why the answer on supplements is clear.

6. What Are Nutrients?

They're more than vitamins, though people often think they are the same thing.

Six important nutrients

Carbohydrates, proteins (which are made up of amino acids*), fats, minerals, vitamins, and water are all nutrients—absorbable components of foods—and necessary for good health. Nutrients are necessary for energy, organ function, food utilization, and cell growth.

7. The Difference Between Micronutrients and Macronutrients

Micronutrients, like vitamins and minerals, do not themselves provide energy. The macronutrients—carbohydrates, fat, and protein—do that, but only when there are sufficient micronutrients to release them.

With nutrients, *less* is often the
same as *more*.

The amount of micronutrients and macronutrients you need for proper health is vastly different—but each is important. (See section 70, "The Protein–Amino Acid Connection.")

*See sections 75–83,

8. How Nutrients Get to Work

> The body simplifies nutrients in
> order to utilize them.

Nutrients basically work through digestion. Digestion is a process of continuous chemical simplification of materials that enter the body through the mouth. Materials are split by enzymatic action into smaller and simpler chemical fragments, which can then be absorbed through the walls of the digestive tract—an open-ended muscular tube, more than thirty feet long, which passes through the body—and finally enter the bloodstream.

9. Understanding Your Digestive System

Knowing how your digestive system works will clear up, right at the start, some of the more common confusions about how, when, and where nutrients operate.

Mouth and Esophagus

Digestion begins in the mouth with the grinding of food and admixture of saliva. An enzyme called ptyalin in the saliva already begins to split starches into simple sugars. The food is then forced to the back of the mouth and into the esophagus, or gullet. Here is where peristalsis begins. This is a kneading "milking" constriction and relaxation of muscles that propels material through the digestive system. To prevent backflow of materials, and to time the release of proper enzymes—since one enzyme cannot do another enzyme's work—the digestive tract is equipped with valves at important junctions.

Stomach

This is the biggest bulge in the digestive tract, as most of us are well aware. But it is located higher than you might think, lying mainly behind the lower ribs, not under the navel, and it does not occupy the belly. It is a flexible bag enclosed by restless muscles, constantly changing form.

• Virtually nothing is absorbed through the stomach walls except alcohol.

> An ordinary meal leaves the stomach
> in three to five hours.

Watery substances, such as soup, leave the stomach quite rapidly. Fats remain considerably longer. An ordinary meal of carbohydrates, proteins, and fats is emptied from the average stomach in *three* to *five* hours. Stomach glands and specialized cells produce mucus, enzymes, hydrochloric acid, and a factor that enables vitamin B_{12} to be dissolved through intestinal walls into the circulation. A normal stomach is definitely on the acid side, and gastric juice, the stomach's special blend, consists of many substances:

Pepsin   The predominant stomach enzyme, a potent digester of meats and other proteins. It is active only in an acid medium.

Renin   Curdles milk.

HCl (Hydrochloric acid)   Produced by stomach cells and creates an acidic state.

The stomach is not absolutely indispensable to digestion. Most of the process of digestion occurs beyond it.

Small Intestine

> Virtually all absorption of nutrients
> occurs in the small intestine.

Twenty-two feet long, here is where digestion is completed and virtually all absorption of nutrients occurs. It has an alkaline environment, brought about by highly alkaline bile, pancreatic juice, and secretions of the intestinal walls. The alkaline environment is necessary for the most important work of digestion and absorption. The *duodenum*, which begins at the stomach outlet, is the first part of the small intestine. This joins with the *jejunum* (about ten feet long), which joins with the *ileum* (ten to twelve feet long). When semiliquid contents of the small intestine are moved along by peristaltic action, we often say we hear our stomach "talking." Actually our stomach lies above these rumblings (called borborygmi), but even with the truth known it's doubtful the phrase will change.

Large Intestine (Colon)

> It takes twelve to fourteen hours for
> contents to make the circuit of the
> large intestine.

Any material leaving the ileum and entering the cecum (where the small and large intestines join) is quite watery. Backflow is prevented at this junction by a muscular valve.

Very little is absorbed from the large intestine except water.

The colon is primarily a storage and dehydrating organ. Substances entering in a liquid state become semisolid as water is absorbed. It takes twelve to fourteen hours for contents to make the circuit of the intestine.

The colon, in contrast to the germ-free stomach, is lavishly populated with bacteria, normal intestinal flora. A large part of the feces is composed of bacteria, along with indigestible material, chiefly cellulose, and substances eliminated from the blood and shed from the intestinal walls.

Liver

The main storage organ for
fat-soluble vitamins.

The liver is the largest solid organ of the body and weighs about four pounds. It is an incomparable chemical plant. It can modify almost any chemical structure. It is a powerful detoxifying organ, breaking down a variety of toxic molecules and rendering them harmless. It is also a blood reservoir and a storage organ for vitamins such as A and D and for digested carbohydrate (glycogen), which is released to sustain blood sugar levels. It manufactures enzymes, cholesterol, proteins, vitamin A (from carotene), and blood coagulation factors.

One of the prime functions of the liver is to produce bile. Bile contains salts that promote efficient digestion of fats by detergent action, emulsifying fatty materials.

Gallbladder

> Even the sight of food may empty
> the gallbladder.

This is a saclike storage organ about three inches long. It holds bile, modifies it chemically, and concentrates it tenfold. The taste or sometimes even the sight of food may be sufficient to empty it out. Constituents of gallbladder fluids sometimes crystallize and form gallstones.

Pancreas

> The pancreas provides the body's most
> important enzymes.

This gland is about six inches long and is nestled into the curve of the duodenum. Its cell clusters secrete insulin, which accelerates the burning of sugar in the body. Insulin is secreted into the blood, not the digestive tract. The larger part of the pancreas manufactures and secretes pancreatic juice, which contains some of the body's most important digestive enzymes—*lipases,* which split fats; *proteases,* which split protein; and *amylases,* which split starches.

10. Name That Vitamin

Because at one time no one knew the chemical structure of vitamins and therefore could not give them a proper scientific name, most are designated by a letter of the alphabet. The following vitamins are known today; many more have yet to be discovered.

Known vitamins from A to U

Vitamin A (retinol, carotene); vitamin B-complex group: B_1 (thiamine), B_2 (riboflavin), B_3 (niacin, niacinamide), B_4 (adenine), B_5 (pantothenic acid), B_6 (pyridoxine), B_{10}, B_{11} (growth factors), B_{12} (cobalamin, cyanocobalamin), B_{13} (orotic acid), B_{15} (pangamic acid), B_{17} (amygdalin), B_c (folic acid), B_T (carnitine), B_x or PABA (para-aminobenzoic acid); choline; inositol; C (ascorbic acid); D (calciferol, viosterol, ergosterol); E (tocopherol); F (fatty acids); G (riboflavin); H (biotin); K (menadione); L (necessary for lactation); M (folic acid); P (bioflavonoids); PP (niacinamide); P_4 (troxerutin); T (growth-promoting substances); U (extracted from cabbage juice).

11. Name That Mineral

The top six minerals are calcium, iodine, iron, magnesium, phosphorus, and zinc.

Although about eighteen known minerals are required for body maintenance and regulatory functions, Recommended Daily Dietary Allowances (RDA) have only been established for six—calcium, iodine, iron, magnesium, phosphorus, and zinc.

The active minerals in your body are calcium, chlorine, chromium, cobalt, copper, fluorine, iodine, iron, magnesium, manganese, molybdenum, phosphorus, potassium, selenium, sodium, sulfur, vanadium, and zinc.

12. Your Body Needs Togetherness

> Vitamins alone are not enough.

As important as vitamins are, they can do nothing for you without minerals. I like to call minerals the Cinderellas of the nutrition world, because, though very few people are aware of it, vitamins cannot function, cannot be assimilated, without the aid of minerals. And though the body can synthesize some vitamins, it cannot manufacture a *single* mineral.

13. Eye-Opening Nutrition Facts

• One cigarette destroys 25–100 mg. of vitamin C!
• Milk with synthetic vitamin D (which means almost all store-bought milk) can rob the body of magnesium!
• People who live in smoggy cities are not getting the vitamin D that their country cousins get because the smog absorbs the sun's ultraviolet rays!
• Daily "happy hours" of more than one cocktail can cause a depletion of vitamins B_1, B_6, and folic acid!
• Eighty percent of American women are deficient in calcium!
• Ten million American women take oral contraceptives and most of them are unaware that the pills can interfere with the availability of vitamins B_6, B_{12}, folic acid, and vitamin C!
• American men rank thirteenth in world health, American women sixth!

• Children need one and a half to two times more protein per pound of body weight than adults—and babies need three times more!

• Cancer researchers at the Massachusetts Institute of Technology have found that vitamins C and E and certain chemicals called *indoles,* found in cabbage, Brussels sprouts, and related vegetables in the crucifer family, are potent and apparently safe inhibitors of certain carcinogens!

• Vitamin B_1 can help fight air- and seasickness.

• If you're on a high-protein diet, your need for B_6 *increases*!

• Onions, garlic, radishes, and leeks all contain a natural antibiotic called *allicin,* which can destroy disease germs without sweeping away the friendly bacteria in the process!

• Aspirin can triple the rate of excretion of your vitamin C!

• Eighteen pecan halves can furnish an entire day's supply of vitamin F!

14. Any Questions About Chapter I?

I've seen quite a few amino acid supplements in health-food stores lately. Are these considered nutrients? Are they as important as vitamins?

Emphatically yes, and yes again! Amino acids (see sections 70 and 75) are the building blocks of one of our most important nutrients—protein.

Every cell in your body contains (and needs) protein. It's used to build new tissue and repair damaged cells, as well as to make hormones and enzymes, keep the acid-alkaline blood content balanced, and eliminate the unwanted garbage, among other things. As protein is digested, it's broken down into smaller compounds called amino acids. When these amino acids reach the cells in your body, they're formed into protein again. It's a wonderful cycle.

The importance of vitamins and amino acids in nutrition is equal, because you'll get no value from one without the proper amount of the other. As for amino acid supplements and their value to you as an individual, I'd suggest looking over sections 75–83, which discuss some of the remarkable benefits supplementation has been shown to provide.

I've learned that the National Institute for Occupational Safety and Health (NIOSH) estimates that one out of every four workers is exposed to substances considered hazardous. What are these jobs, and what supplements should these workers be taking?

I couldn't name all of the jobs, but the following is a list of some:

Electrical engineers, electricians, and printers Exposure to electronic devices, fluorescent lights, disinfectants, measuring devices, or certain dyes and inks may subject you to an odorless mercury that can cause emotional disorders or even death.

Secretaries and receptionists Certain duplicating machines give off fumes that may cause visual problems, fatigue, and headaches. Some switchboards can release ozone, a colorless vapor that may cause respiratory disorders.

Paperhangers There are wallpapers coated with vinyl chloride, apparently carcinogenic, a chemical that can easily be inhaled.

Dentists, dental hygienists   The silver amalgam, often used for fillings, contains mercury and can give off vapors. The Institute for Occupational Safety estimates that there are unhealthy levels of mercury in one out of every ten dentists' offices.

Mechanics   If you work with machinery that is cleaned with solvents, you can inhale vapors that may be injurious to your health, causing skin inflammations as well as liver and kidney disturbances.

Asbestos workers   It is estimated that 45 percent of asbestos-insulation workers will die of some form of cancer. (Breathing in buildings where asbestos has been sprayed on steel beams and may flake off could be dangerous to anyone's health.)

Workers in any of these occupations should be taking supplemental antioxidants daily: vitamins A, C, E, and selenium!

II

A Vitamin Pill Is a Vitamin Pill Is a...

15. Where Vitamins Come From

> Most vitamins are extracted from
> basic natural sources.

Because vitamins are natural substances found in foods, the supplements you take—be they capsules, tablets, powers, or liquids—also come from foods. Though many of the vitamins can be synthesized, most are extracted from basic natural sources.

For example: Vitamin A usually comes from fish liver oil. Vitamin B complex comes from yeast or liver. Vitamin C is best when derived from rose hips, the berries found on the fruit of the rose after the petals have fallen off. And vitamin E is generally extracted from soybeans, wheat germ, or corn.

16. Why Vitamins Come in Different Forms

Everyone's needs are different, and for this reason manufacturers have provided many vitamins in a variety of forms.

Vitamins come in different forms
because people do.

Tablets are the most common and convenient form. They're easier to store, carry, and have a longer shelf life than powders or liquids.

Capsules, like tablets, are convenient and easy to store, and are the usual supplement for oil-soluble vitamins such as A, D, and E.

Powders have advantages of extra potency (1 tsp. of many vitamin-C powders can give you as much as 4,000 mg.) and the added benefit of no fillers, binders, or additives for anyone with allergies.

Liquids are available for easy mixing with beverages and for people unable to swallow capsules and tablets.

17. Oil vs. Dry or Water Soluble

The oil-soluble vitamins, such as A, D, E, and K, are available and advisable in "dry" or water-soluble form for people who tend to get upset stomachs from oil, for acne sufferers or anyone with a skin condition where oil ingestion is not advised, and for dieters who have cut most of the fat from their meals. (Fat-soluble vitamins need fat for proper assimilation. If you're on a low-fat diet and taking A, D, E, or K supplements, I suggest you use the dry form.)

18. Synthetic vs. Natural and Inorganic vs. Organic

> Synthetic vitamins might be less
> likely to upset your budget—
> but not your stomach.

When I'm asked if there's a difference between synthetic and natural vitamins, I usually say only one—and that's to you. Though synthetic vitamins and minerals have produced satisfactory results, the benefits from natural vitamins, on a variety of levels, surpass them. Chemical analysis of both might appear the same, but there's more to natural vitamins because there's more to those substances in nature.

Synthetic vitamin C is just that: ascorbic acid, and nothing more. Natural C from rose hips contains bioflavonoids, the entire C complex, which make the C much more effective.

Natural vitamin E, which can include all the tocopherols, not just alpha, is more potent than its synthetic double.

According to Dr. Theron G. Randolph, noted allergist:

A synthetically derived substance may cause a reaction in a chemically susceptible person when the same material of natural origin is tolerated, despite the two substances having identical chemical structures.

On the other hand, people who are allergic to pollen could experience an undesirable reaction to a natural vitamin C that had possible pollen impurities.

Nonetheless, as many who have tried both can attest, there are less gastrointestinal upsets with natural supplements and far fewer toxic reactions when taken in higher than recommended dosage.

The difference between inorganic and organic is not the same as the one between synthetic and natural, though that is the common misconception. All vitamins are organic. They are substances containing carbon.

19. Chelation, And What It Means

> Only 2 to 10 percent of inorganic iron taken into the body is actually absorbed.

First, pronounce it correctly. *Key'lation*. This is the process by which mineral substances are changed into their digestible form. Common mineral supplements such as bonemeal and dolomite are often not chelated and must first be acted upon in the digestive process to form chelates before they are of use to the body. The natural chelating process is not performed efficiently in many people, and because of this a good deal of the mineral supplements they take is of little use.

When you realize that the body does not use whatever it takes in, that most of us do not digest our foods efficiently, that only 2 to 10 percent of inorganic iron taken into the body is actually absorbed, and, even with this small percentage, 50 percent is then eliminated, you can recognize the importance of taking minerals that have been chelated. Amino acid–bound chelated mineral supplements provide three to ten times greater assimilation than the nonchelated ones, and are well worth the small additional cost.

20. Time Release

A major step forward in vitamin manufacturing has been the introduction of time-release supplements. Time release is a process by which vitamins are enrobed in micropellets (tiny time pills) and then combined into a special base for their release in a pattern that assures six- to twelve-hour absorption. Most vitamins are water soluble and cannot be stored in the body. Without time release, they are quickly absorbed into the bloodstream and, no matter how large the dose, are excreted in the urine within two to three hours.

> A way to twenty-four-hour vitamin
> protection.

Time-release supplements can offer optimum effectiveness, minimal excretory loss, and stable blood levels all during the day and through the night.

21. Fillers, Binders, Or What Else Am I Getting?

There's more to a vitamin supplement than meets the eye— and sometimes more than meets the label. Fillers, binders, lubricants, and the like do not have to be listed and often aren't. But if you'd like to know what you're swallowing, the following list should help.

Diluents or fillers These are inert materials added to the tablets to increase their bulk, in order to make them a practical size for compression. Dicalcium phosphate, which is an excellent source of calcium and phosphorus, is used in better brands. It is a white powder derived from purified mineral rocks. Sorbitol and cellulose (plant fiber) are used occasionally.

Binders   These substances give cohesive qualities to the powdered materials, otherwise the binders or granulators are the materials that hold the ingredients of the tablet together. Cellulose and ethyl cellulose are used most often. Cellulose is the main constituent of plant fiber. Other binders that can be used are:

acacia (gum arabic)—a vegetable gum
algin—alginic acid or sodium alginate—a plant carbohydrate derived from seaweed
lecithin and sorbitol (used occasionally)

Lubricants   A slick substance added to a tablet to keep it from sticking to the machines that punch it out. Calcium stearate and silica are commonly used. Calcium stearate is derived from natural vegetable oils. Silica is a natural white powder. Magnesium stearate can also be used.

Disintegrators   Substances such as gum arabic, algin, and alginate are added to the tablet to facilitate its breakup or disintegration after ingestion.

Colors   They make the tablet more aesthetic or elegant in appearance. Colors derived from natural sources, like chlorophyll, are best.

Flavors and sweeteners   Used only in chewable tablets, the sweeteners are usually fructose (fruit sugar), malt dextrins, sorbitol, or maltose. Sucrose (sugar) is rarely used in better brands.

Coating materials   These substances are used to protect the tablet from moisture. They also mask unpleasant flavor or odor and make the tablet easier to swallow. Zein is one of the substances. It is natural, derived from corn protein, and a clear film-coating agent. Brazil wax, which is a natural product derived from palm trees, is also frequently used.

Drying agents   These substances prevent water-absorbing (hydroscopic) materials from picking up moisture during processing. Silica gel is the most common drying agent.

22. Storage and Staying Power

Vitamin and mineral supplements should be stored in a cool dark place away from direct sunlight in a well-closed—preferably opaque—container. They do not have to be stored in the refrigerator unless you live in a desert climate. To guard against excessive moisture, place a few kernels of rice at the bottom of your vitamin bottle. The rice works as a natural absorbent.

Vitamins can last two to three years
in a well-sealed container.

If vitamins are kept cool and away from light, and remain well sealed, they should last for two to three years. To insure freshness, though, your best bet is to buy brands that have an expiration date on the label. Once a bottle is opened you can expect a twelve-month shelf life.

Our bodies tend to excrete in urine substances we take in on a four-hour basis, and this is particularly true of water-soluble vitamins such as B and C. On an empty stomach, B and C vitamins can leave the body as quickly as two hours after ingestion.

The oil-soluble vitamins, A, D, E, and K, remain in

the body for approximately twenty-four hours, though excess amounts can be stored in the liver for much longer. Dry A and E do not stay in the body as long.

23. When and How to Take Supplements

The human body operates on a twenty-four-hour cycle. Your cells do not go to sleep when you do, nor can they exist without continuous oxygen and nutrients. Therefore, for best results, space your supplements as evenly as possible during the day.

> If you take your supplements all
> at once, do so after dinner,
> not breakfast.

The prime time for taking supplements is after meals. Vitamins are organic substances and should be taken with other foods and minerals for best absorption. Because the water-soluble vitamins, especially B complex and C, are excreted fairly rapidly in the urine, a regimen of after breakfast, after lunch, and after dinner will provide you with the highest body level. If after each meal is not convenient, then half the amount should be taken after breakfast and the other half after dinner.

If you must take your vitamins all at once, then do so after the largest meal of the day. In other words, for best results, after dinner, not after breakfast, is the most desirable.

And remember, minerals are essential for proper vitamin absorption, so be sure to take your minerals and vitamins together.

24. What's Right for You

If you're unsure as to whether you'd be better off with a powder, a liquid, or a tablet, regular vitamin E or dry, taking supplements three times a day or time released, my advice to you is to experiment. If the supplement you're taking doesn't agree with you, try it in another form. Vitamin-C powder mixed in a beverage might be much easier to take than several large pills when you're coming down with a cold. If your face breaks out with vitamin E, try the dry form. Check sections 26 through 68 and the cautions in section 277 to make sure you know all you should about your supplement.

25. Any Questions About Chapter II?

When vitamins smell awful, does that mean they're spoiled, and could they be harmful?

Strong odors don't necessarily signify spoilage, but it is possible. If you've been keeping your vitamins in sunlight and warmth (great for you but not for them) it's more than possible, it's probable. But even if your vitamins have spoiled, they won't harm you. The worst that can happen is that they lose their effectiveness.

Every so often I detect a sort of alcohol smell in a bottle of vitamins. Does this indicate some sort of deterioration, and are these vitamins still safe to take?

No, the vitamins are not deteriorating, and yes, they are safe to take. Alcohol is often used as a drying agent to prevent any moisture contamination. Occasionally, if the product is packed too quickly, some of the alcohol smell remains. My advice is put a few kernels of rice in the bottle. These will absorb the moisture and the smell.

Sometimes I find that a few of my B vitamin pills are cracked. Are these safe to take?

Yes, they are, as are your C's and any others. Poor tablet coating causes the cracks, but the vitamins themselves are still effective and safe.

III

Everything You Always Wanted to Know About Vitamins but Had No One to Ask

26. Vitamin A

FACTS:

Vitamin A is fat soluble. It requires fats as well as minerals to be properly absorbed by your digestive tract.

It can be stored in your body and need not be replenished every day.

It occurs in two forms—preformed vitamin A, called retinol (found only in foods of animal origin), and provitamin A, known as carotene (provided by foods of both plant and animal origin).

Vitamin A is measured in USP units (United States Pharmacopeia), IU (international units), and—most recently— RE (retinol equivalents). (See section 124.)

A daily dosage of 1,000 RE (or 5,000 IU) is recommended for adult males to prevent deficiency. For females it's 800 RE (4,000 IU). During pregnancy an additional 200 RE (1,000 IU) is required, and for nursing mothers an additional 400 RE (2,000 IU) is recommended.

WHAT IT CAN DO FOR YOU:

Counteract night blindness, weak eyesight, and aid in the treatment of many eye disorders. (It permits formation of visual purple in the eye.)

Build resistance to respiratory infections.

Shorten the duration of diseases.

Keep the outer layers of your tissues and organs healthy.

Help in the removal of age spots.

Promote growth, strong bones, healthy skin, hair, teeth, and gums.

Help treat acne, impetigo, boils, carbuncles, and open ulcers when applied externally.

Aid in the treatment of emphysema and hyperthyroidism.

DEFICIENCY DISEASE:

Xerophthalmia, night blindness. (For deficiency symptoms, see section 119.)

BEST NATURAL SOURCES:

Fish liver oil, liver, carrots, green and yellow vegetables, eggs, milk and dairy products, margarine, and yellow fruits.

SUPPLEMENTS:

Usually available in two forms, one derived from natural fish liver oil and the other water dispersible.

Water-dispersible supplements are either acetate or palmitate and are recommended for anyone intolerant to oil, particularly acne sufferers.

Vitamin A acid (retin A) is sometimes prescribed for acne but is available only by prescription. The most common daily doses are 10,000 to 25,000 IU.

TOXICITY:

More than 100,000 IU daily can produce toxic effects in adults, if taken for many months.

More than 18,500 IU daily can produce toxic effects in infants (one cup of cooked, diced carrots contains 15,000 IU vitamin A.)

Toxicity symptoms include hair loss, nausea, vomiting, diarrhea, scaly skin, blurred vision, rashes, bone pain, irregular menses, fatigue, headaches, and liver enlargement. (See section 277, "Cautions.")

ENEMIES:

Polyunsaturated fatty acids with carotene work against vitamin A unless there are antioxidants present. (See section 49 for antioxidants, and section 239 for drugs that deplete vitamins.)

PERSONAL ADVICE:

You need at least 10,000 IU vitamin A if you take more than 400 IU vitamin E daily.

If you are on the pill, your need for A is *decreased*.

If your weekly diet includes ample amounts of liver, carrots, spinach, sweet potatoes, or cantaloupe, it's unlikely you need an A supplement.

Vitamin A should *not* be taken with mineral oil.

Vitamin A works best with B complex, vitamin D, vitamin E, calcium, phosphorus, and zinc. (Zinc is what's needed by the liver to get vitamin A out of its storage deposits.)

Vitamin A also helps vitamin C from oxidizing.

Don't supplement your dog's or cat's diet with vitamin A unless a vet specifically advises it.

If you are on a cholesterol-reducing drug such as Questran (cholestyramine), you'll have decreased vitamin A absorption and probably need a supplement.

To prevent buildup in system, take supplement for only 5 days a week—then stop for 2.

27. Vitamin B₁ (Thiamine)

FACTS:

Water soluble. Like all the B-complex vitamins, any excess is excreted and not stored in the body. It must be replaced daily.

Measured in milligrams (mg.).

Being synergistic, B vitamins are more potent together than when used separately. B_1, B_2, and B_6 should be equally balanced (i.e., 50 mg. of B_1, 50 mg. of B_2, and 50 mg. of B_6) to work effectively.

The official RDA for adults is 1.0 to 1.5 mg. (During pregnancy and lactation 1.4 to 1.6 mg. is suggested.)

Need increases during illness, stress, and surgery.

Known as the "morale vitamin" because of its beneficial effects on the nervous system and mental attitude.

Has a mild diuretic effect.

WHAT IT CAN DO FOR YOU:

Promote growth.
Aid digestion, especially of carbohydrates.
Improve your mental attitude.
Keep nervous system, muscles, and heart functioning normally.
Help fight air- or seasickness.
Relieve dental postoperative pain.
Aid in treatment of herpes zoster.

DEFICIENCY DISEASE:

Beriberi. (For deficiency symptoms, see section 119.)

BEST NATURAL SOURCES:

Dried yeast, rice husks, whole wheat, oatmeal, peanuts, pork, most vegetables, bran, milk.

SUPPLEMENTS:

Available in low- and high-potency dosages—usually 50 mg., 100 mg., and 500 mg. It is most effective in B-complex formulas, balanced with B_2 and B_6. It is even more effective when the formula contains antistress pantothenic acid, folic acid, and B_{12}. The most common daily doses are 100 to 300 mg.

TOXICITY:

No known toxicity for this water-soluble vitamin. Any excess is excreted in the urine and not stored to any degree in tissues or organs.

Rare excess symptoms include tremors, herpes, edema, nervousness, rapid heartbeat, and allergies.

(See section 277, "Cautions.")

ENEMIES:

Cooking heat easily destroys this B vitamin. Other enemies of B_1 are caffeine, alcohol, food-processing methods, air, water, estrogen, antacids, and sulfa drugs. (See section 239 for drugs that deplete vitamins.)

PERSONAL ADVICE:

If you are a smoker, drinker, or heavy sugar consumer, you need more vitamin B_1.

If you are pregnant, nursing, or on the pill, you have a greater need for this vitamin.

If you're in the habit of taking an after-dinner antacid, you're losing the thiamine you might have gotten from the meal.

As with all stress conditions—disease, anxiety, trauma, postsurgery—your B-complex intake, which includes thiamine, should be increased.

28. Vitamin B_2 (Riboflavin)

FACTS:

Water soluble. Easily absorbed. The amount excreted depends on bodily needs and may be accompanied by protein loss. Like the other B vitamins, it is not stored and must be replaced regularly through whole foods or supplements.

Also known as vitamin G.

Measured in milligrams (mg.).

Unlike thiamine, riboflavin is *not* destroyed by heat, oxidation, or acid.

For normal adults, 1.2 to 1.7 mg. is the RDA. Slightly higher amounts are suggested during pregnancy and lactation.

Increased need in stress situations.

America's most common vitamin deficiency is riboflavin.

WHAT IT CAN DO FOR YOU:

Aid in growth and reproduction.

Promote healthy skin, nails, and hair.

Help eliminate sore mouth, lips, and tongue.

Benefit vision, alleviate eye fatigue.

Function with other substances to metabolize carbohydrates, fats, and proteins.

DEFICIENCY DISEASE:

Ariboflavinosis—mouth, lips, skin, and genitalia lesions. (For deficiency symptoms, see section 119.)

BEST NATURAL SOURCES:

Milk, liver, kidney, yeast, cheese, leafy green vegetables, fish, eggs.

SUPPLEMENTS:

Available in both low and high potencies—most commonly in 100-mg. doses. Like most of the B-complex vitamins, it is most effective when in a well-balanced formula with the others.

The most common daily doses are 100 to 300 mg.

TOXICITY:

No known toxic effects.

Possible symptoms of minor excess include itching, numbness, sensations of burning or prickling.

(See section 277, "Cautions.")

ENEMIES:

Light—especially ultraviolet light—and alkalies are destructive to riboflavin. (Opaque milk cartons now protect riboflavin that used to be destroyed in clear glass milk bottles.) Other natural enemies are water (B_2 dissolves in cooking liquids), sulfa drugs, estrogen, and alcohol.

PERSONAL ADVICE:

If you are taking the pill, pregnant, or lactating, you need more vitamin B_2.

If you eat little red meat or dairy products you should increase your intake.

There is a strong likelihood of your being deficient in this vitamin if you are on a prolonged restricted diet for ulcers or diabetes. (In all cases where you are under medical treatment for a specific illness, check with your doctor before altering your present food regimen or embarking on a new one.)

All stress conditions require additional B complex.

This vitamin works best with vitamin B_6, vitamin C, and niacin.

If you're taking an antineoplastic (anticancer) drug such as methotrexate, too much vitamin B_2 can cut down the drug's effectiveness.

29. Vitamin B_6 (Pyridoxine)

FACTS:

Water soluble. Excreted within eight hours after ingestion and, like the other B vitamins, needs to be replaced by whole foods or supplements.

B_6 is actually a group of substances—pyridoxine, pyridoxinal, and pyridoxamine—that are closely related and function together.

Measured in milligrams (mg.).

Requirement increased when high-protein diets are consumed.

Must be present for the production of antibodies and red blood cells.

There is some evidence of synthesis by intestinal bacteria, and that a vegetable diet supplemented with cellulose is responsible.

The recommended adult intake is 1.8 to 2.2 mg. daily, with higher doses suggested during pregnancy and lactation.

Required for the proper absorption of vitamin B_{12}.

Necessary for the production of hydrochloric acid and magnesium.

WHAT IT CAN DO FOR YOU:

Properly assimilate protein and fat.

Aid in the conversion of tryptophan, an essential amino acid, to niacin.

Help prevent various nervous and skin disorders.

Alleviate nausea (many morning-sickness preparations that doctors prescribe include vitamin B_6).

Promote proper synthesis of antiaging nucleic acids.

Help reduce dry mouth and urination problems caused by tricyclic antidepressants.

Reduce night muscle spasms, leg cramps, hand numbness, certain forms of neuritis in the extremities.

Work as a natural diuretic.

DEFICIENCY DISEASE:

Anemia, seborrheic dermatitis, glossitis. (For deficiency symptoms, see section 119.)

BEST NATURAL SOURCES:

Brewer's yeast, wheat bran, wheat germ, liver, kidney, heart, cantaloupe, cabbage, blackstrap molasses, milk, eggs, beef.

SUPPLEMENTS:

Readily available in a wide range of dosages—from 50 to 500 mg.—in individual supplements as well as in B-complex and multivitamin formulas.

To prevent deficiencies in other B vitamins, pyridoxine should be taken in equal amounts with B_1 and B_2.

Can be purchased in time-disintegrating formulas that provide for gradual release up to ten hours.

TOXICITY:

Daily doses of 2 to 10 grams can cause neurological disorders.

Possible symptom of an oversupply of B_6 is night restlessness and too vivid dream recall.

Doses over 500 mg. are not recommended. (See section 277, "Cautions.")

ENEMIES:

Long storage, canning, roasting or stewing of meat, water, food-processing techniques, alcohol, estrogen. (See section 239.)

PERSONAL ADVICE:

If you are on the pill, you are more than likely to need increased amounts of B_6.

Heavy protein consumers need extra amounts of this vitamin.

Vitamin B_6 might decrease a diabetic's requirement for insulin, and if the dosage is not adjusted, a low-blood-sugar reaction could result.

Arthritis sufferers being treated with Cuprimine (penicillamine) should be taking supplements of this vitamin.

This vitamin works best with vitamin B_1, vitamin B_2, pantothenic acid, vitamin C, and magnesium.

Supplements for this vitamin should *not* be taken by anyone under levodopa treatment for Parkinson's disease!

(Ask your doctor about Sinemet, a drug that can bypass this particular adverse vitamin interaction.)

30. Vitamin B_{12} (Cobalamin)

FACTS:

Water soluble and effective in very small doses.

Commonly known as the "red vitamin," also cyano-cobalamin.

Measured in micrograms (mcg.).

The only vitamin that contains essential mineral elements.

Not well assimilated through the stomach. Needs to be combined with calcium during absorption to properly benefit body.

Recommended adult dose is 3 mcg., with larger amounts suggested for pregnant and lactating women.

A diet low in B_1 and high in folic acid (such as a vegetarian diet) often hides a vitamin-B_{12} deficiency.

A properly functioning thyroid gland helps B_{12} absorption. Symptoms of B_{12} deficiency may take more than five years to appear after body stores have been depleted.

WHAT IT CAN DO FOR YOU:

Form and regenerate red blood cells, thereby preventing anemia.

Promote growth and increase appetite in children.

Increase energy.

Maintain a healthy nervous system.

Properly utilize fats, carbohydrates, and protein.

Relieve irritability.

Improve concentration, memory, and balance.

DEFICIENCY DISEASE:

Pernicious anemia, brain damage. (For deficiency symptoms, see section 119.)

BEST NATURAL SOURCES:

Liver, beef, pork, eggs, milk, cheese, kidney.

SUPPLEMENTS:

Because B_{12} is not absorbed well through the stomach, I recommend the sublingual form of the vitamin, or the time-release form—accompanied by sorbitol—so that it can be assimilated in the small intestine.

Supplements are available in a variety of strengths from 50 to 2,000 mcg.

Doctors routinely give vitamin-B_{12} injections. If there is a severe indication of deficiency or extreme fatigue, this method might be the supplementation that's called for.

Daily doses most often used are 5 to 100 mcg.

TOXICITY:

There have been no cases reported of vitamin-B_{12} toxicity, even on megadose regimens.

(See section 277, "Cautions.")

ENEMIES:

Acids and alkalies, water, sunlight, alcohol, estrogen, sleeping pills. (See section 239.)

PERSONAL ADVICE:

If you are a vegetarian and have excluded eggs and dairy products from your diet, than you need B_{12} supplementation.

If you keep regular "Happy Hours" and drink a lot, B_{12} is an important supplement for you.

Combined with folic acid, B_{12} can be a most effective revitalizer.

Surprisingly, heavy protein consumers may also need extra amounts of this vitamin, which works synergistically with almost all other B vitamins as well as vitamins A, E, and C.

Women may find B_{12} helpful—as part of a B complex—during and just prior to menstruation.

31. Vitamin B_{13} (Orotic Acid)

FACTS:

Not readily available alone in the United States but can be obtained in combination with minerals.

Metabolizes folic acid and vitamin B_{12}.

No RDA has been established.

WHAT IT CAN DO FOR YOU:

Possibly prevent certain liver problems and premature aging.

Aid in the treatment of multiple sclerosis.

DEFICIENCY DISEASE:

Deficiency symptoms and diseases related to this vitamin are still uncertain.

BEST NATURAL SOURCES:

Root vegetables, whey, the liquid portion of soured or curdled milk.

SUPPLEMENTS:

Available as calcium orotate in supplemental form.

TOXICITY:

Too little is known about the vitamin at this time to establish guidelines.

(See section 277, "Cautions.")

ENEMIES:

Water and sunlight.

PERSONAL ADVICE:

Not enough research has been done on this vitamin for recommendations to be made.

32. B₁₅ (Pangamic Acid)

FACTS:

Water soluble.
Because its essential requirement for diet has not been proved, it is not a vitamin in the strict sense.
Measured in milligrams (mg.).
Works much like vitamin E in that it is an antioxidant.
Introduced by the Russians, who are thrilled with its results; the U.S. Food and Drug Administration has taken it off the market in its pangamic acid and calcium pangamic form.
Action is often improved when taken with vitamin A and E.

WHAT IT CAN DO FOR YOU:*

Extend cell life span.
Neutralize the craving for liquor.
Speed recovery from fatigue.
Lower blood cholesterol levels.
Protect against pollutants.
Relieve symptoms of angina and asthma.
Protect the liver against cirrhosis.
Ward off hangovers.
Stimulate immunity responses.
Aid in protein synthesis.

*U.S. research in the case of B₁₅ has been limited. The list of benefits given here is based on my study of Soviet tests.

DEFICIENCY DISEASE:

Again, research has been limited, but indications point to glandular and nerve disorders, heart disease, and diminished oxygenation of living tissue.

BEST NATURAL SOURCES:

Brewer's yeast, whole brown rice, whole grains, pumpkin seeds, sesame seeds.

SUPPLEMENTS:

Usually available in 50-mg. strengths.
Daily doses most often used are 50 to 150 mgs.

TOXICITY:

There have been no reported cases of toxicity. Some people say they have experienced nausea on beginning a B_{15} regimen, but this usually disappears after a few days and can be alleviated by taking the B_{15} supplement after the day's largest meal.
(See section 277, "Cautions.")

ENEMIES:

Water and sunlight.

PERSONAL ADVICE:

Despite the controversy, I have found B_{15} effective and believe most diets would benefit from supplementation.

(Dr. Atkins prescribes it for anyone on his super-energy diet.)

If you are an athlete or just want to feel like one, I suggest one 50-mg. tablet in the morning with breakfast and one in the evening with dinner.

An important supplement for residents of big cities and high-density pollution areas.

33. Vitamin B$_{17}$ (Laetrile)

FACTS:

One of the most controversial "vitamins" of the decade.

Chemically a compound of two sugar molecules (one benzaldehyde and one cyanide) called an amygdalin.

Known as nitrilosides when used in medical doses.

Made from apricot pits.

One B vitamin that is not present in brewer's yeast.

Unaccepted as a cancer treatment in most of the United States at this date. (Legal in twenty-four states.) Rejected by the Food and Drug Administration on the grounds it might be poisonous due to its cyanide content.

WHAT IT CAN DO FOR YOU:

It is purported to have specific cancer-controlling and preventive properties.

DEFICIENCY DISEASE:

May lead to diminished resistance to cancer.

BEST NATURAL SOURCES:

A small amount of laetrile is found in the whole kernels of apricots, apples, cherries, peaches, plums, nectarines.

SUPPLEMENTS:

Daily doses most often used are 0.25 to 1.0 g.

TOXICITY:

Though no toxicity levels have been established yet, taking excessive amounts of laetrile could be dangerous. Cumulative amounts of more than 3.0 g. can be ingested safety, but not more than 1.0 g. at any one time.

According to the *Nutrition Almanac,* five to thirty apricot kernels eaten throughout the day, but never all at the same time, can be a sufficient preventive amount.

(See section 277, "Cautions.")

PERSONAL ADVICE:

If you are interested in laetrile as a cancer preventive or treatment, check with a nutrition-oriented physician. If you know of none in your area, send a stamped, self-addressed envelope with your query to the International College of Applied Nutrition (P.O. Box 386, La Habra, CA 90631) for a referral.

There is now extensive literature available on laetrile. I strongly advise personal research and a consultation with a physician before embarking on any regimen involving B_{17}.

34. Biotin (Coenzyme R or Vitamin H)

FACTS:

Water soluble, and another fairly recent member of the B-complex family.

Usually measured in micrograms (mcg.).

Synthesis of ascorbic acid requires biotin.

Essential for normal metabolism of fat and protein.

The RDA for adults is 150 to 300 mcg.

Can be synthesized by intestinal bacteria.

Raw eggs prevent absorption by the body.

Synergistic with B_2, B_6, niacin, A, and in maintaining healthy skin.

WHAT IT CAN DO FOR YOU:

Aid in keeping hair from turning gray.

Help in preventive treatment for baldness.

Ease muscle pains.

Alleviate eczema and dermatitis.

DEFICIENCY DISEASE:

Eczema of face and body, extreme exhaustion, impairment of fat metabolism. (For deficiency symptoms, see section 119.)

BEST NATURAL SOURCES:

Nuts, fruits, brewer's yeast, beef liver, egg yolk, milk, kidney, unpolished rice.

SUPPLEMENTS:

Biotin is usually included in most B-complex supplements and multiple-vitamin tablets.

Daily doses most often used are 25 to 300 mcg.

TOXICITY:

There are no known cases of biotin toxicity.
(See section 277, "Cautions.")

ENEMIES:

Raw egg white (which contains avidin, a protein that prevents biotin absorption), water, sulfa drugs, estrogen, food-processing techniques, and alcohol. (See section 239.)

PERSONAL ADVICE:

If you drink a lot of eggnogs made with raw eggs you probably need biotin supplementation.

Be sure you're getting at least 25 mcg. daily if you are on antibiotics or sulfa drugs.

Balding men might find that a biotin supplement may keep their hair there longer.

Keep in mind that biotin works synergistically—and more effectively—with B_2, B_6, niacin, and A.

35. Vitamin C (Ascorbic Acid, Cevitamin Acid)

FACTS:

Water soluble.

Most animals synthesize their own vitamin C, but

man, apes, and guinea pigs must rely upon dietary sources.

Plays a primary role in the formation of collagen, which is important for the growth and repair of body tissue cells, gums, blood vessels, bones, and teeth.

Helps in the body's absorption of iron.

Measured in milligrams (mg.).

Used up more rapidly under stress conditions.

The RDA for adults is 60 mg. (higher doses recommended during pregnancy and lactation—80 to 120 mg.).

Smokers and older persons have greater need for vitamin C. (Each cigarette destroys 25–100 mg.)

Recommended as a preventive for crib death or Sudden Infant Death Syndrome (SIDS).

WHAT IT CAN DO FOR YOU:

Heal wounds, burns, and bleeding gums.

Increase effectiveness of drugs used to treat urinary tract infections.

Accelerate healing after surgery.

Help in decreasing blood cholesterol.

Aid in preventing many types of viral and bacterial infections and generally potentiate the immune system.

Offer protection against cancer-producing agents.

Help counteract the formation of nitrosamines (cancer-causing substances).

Act as a natural laxative.

Lower incidence of blood clots in veins.

Aid in treatment and prevention of the common cold.

Extend life by enabling protein cells to hold together.

Reduce effects of many allergy-producing substances.

Prevent scurvy.

DEFICIENCY DISEASE:

Scurvy. (For deficiency symptoms, see section 119.)

BEST NATURAL SOURCES:

Citrus fruits, berries, green and leafy vegetables, tomatoes, cauliflower, potatoes, sweet potatoes.

SUPPLEMENTS:

Vitamin C is one of the most widely taken supplements. It is available in conventional pills, time-release tablets, syrups, powders, chewable wafers, in just about every form a vitamin can take.

The form that is *pure* vitamin C is derived from corn dextrose (though no corn or dextrose remains).

The difference between "natural" or "organic" vitamin C and ordinary ascorbic acid is primarily in the individual's ability to digest it.

The best vitamin-C supplement is one that contains the complete C complex of bioflavonoids, hesperidin, and rutin. (Sometimes these are labeled citrus salts.)

Tablets and capsules are usually supplied in strengths up to 1,000 mg., and in powder form sometimes 5,000 mg. per tsp.

Daily doses most often used are 500 mg. to 4 g.

Rose hips vitamin C contains bioflavonoids and other enzymes that help C assimilate. They are the richest natural source of vitamin C. (The C is actually manufactured under the bud of the rose—called a hip.)

Acerola C is made with acerola berries.

TOXICITY:

Excessive intake may cause oxalic acid and uric acid stone formation (though taking magnesium, vitamin B_6, and a sufficient amount of water daily can rectify this). Occasionally, very high doses (over 10 g. daily) can cause unpleasant side effects, such as diarrhea, excess urination, and skin rashes. If any of these occur, cut back on your dosage.

Vitamin C should not be used by cancer patients undergoing radiation or chemotherapy.

(See section 277, "Caution.")

ENEMIES:

Water, cooking, heat, light, oxygen, smoking. (See section 239.)

PERSONAL ADVICE:

Because vitamin C is excreted in two to three hours, depending on the quantity of food in the stomach, and it is important to maintain a constant high level of C in the bloodstream at all times, I recommend a time-release tablet for optimal effectiveness.

Large doses of vitamin C can alter the results of laboratory tests. If you're going to have any blood or urine testing, be sure to inform your doctor that you're taking vitamin C so that no errors will be made in diagnosis (vitamin C can mask the presence of blood in stool).

Diabetics should be aware that testing the urine for sugar could be inaccurate if you're taking a lot of vitamin C (but there are testing kits available that aren't affected by vitamin C. Ask your pharmacist or physician).

If you're taking over 750 mg. daily, I suggest a magnesium supplement. This is an effective deterrent against kidney stones.

Carbon monoxide destroys vitamin C, so city dwellers should definitely up their intake.

You need extra C if you are on the pill.

To maximize the effectiveness of vitamin C, remember that it works best in conjunction with bioflavonoids, calcium, and magnesium.

I recommend increasing C doses if you take aspirin, which triples the excretion rate of vitamin C.

If you take ginseng, it's better to take it three hours before or after taking vitamin C or foods that are high in the vitamin.

36. Calcium Pantothenate (Pantothenic Acid, Panthenol, Vitamin B₅)

FACTS:

Water soluble, another member of the B-complex family.

Helps in cell building, maintaining normal growth, and development of the central nervous system.

Vital for the proper functioning of the adrenal glands.

Essential for conversion of fat and sugar to energy.

Necessary for synthesis of antibodies, for utilization of PABA and choline.

The RDA (as set by the FDA) is 10 mg. for adults.

Can be synthesized in the body by intestinal bacteria.

WHAT IT CAN DO FOR YOU:

Aid in wound healing.
Fight infection by building antibodies.
Treat postoperative shock.
Prevent fatigue.
Reduce adverse and toxic effects of many antibiotics.

DEFICIENCY DISEASE:

Hypoglycemia, duodenal ulcers, blood and skin disorders. (For deficiency symptoms, see section 119.)

BEST NATURAL SOURCES:

Meat, whole grains, wheat germ, bran, kidney, liver, heart, green vegetables, brewer's yeast, nuts, chicken, crude molasses.

SUPPLEMENTS:

Most commonly found in B-complex formulas in a variety of strengths from 10 to 100 mg.
The daily doses usually taken are 10 to 300 mg.

TOXICITY:

No known toxic effects.
(See section 277, "Cautions.")

ENEMIES:

Heat, food-processing techniques, canning, caffeine, sulfa drugs, sleeping pills, estrogen, alcohol. (See section 239.)

PERSONAL ADVICE:

If you frequently have tingling hands and feet, you might try increasing your pantothenic acid intake—in combination with other B vitamins.

Pantothenic acid can help provide a defense against a stress situation that you foresee or are involved in.

A daily dosage of 1,000 mg. has been found effective in reducing the pain of arthritis, in some cases.

If you suffer from allergies, relief could be just a vitamin B_5 and C away. Try taking 1,000 mg. of each—with food—morning and evening.

37. Choline

FACTS:

A member of the B-complex family and a lipotropic (fat emulsifier).

Works with inositol (another B-complex member) to utilize fats and cholesterol.

One of the few substances able to penetrate the so-called blood-brain barrier, which ordinarily protects the brain against variations in the daily diet, and go directly into the brain cells to produce a chemical that aids memory.

The RDA has not yet been established, though it's

estimated that the average adult diet contains between 500 and 900 mg. a day.

Seems to emulsify cholesterol so that it doesn't settle on artery walls or in the gallbladder.

WHAT IT CAN DO FOR YOU:

Help control cholesterol buildup.

Aid in the sending of nerve impulses, specifically those in the brain used in the formation of memory.

Assist in conquering the problem of memory loss in later years (doses of 1 to 5 g. a day).

Help eliminate poisons and drugs from your system by aiding the liver.

Produce a soothing effect.

Aid in the treatment of Alzheimer's disease.

DEFICIENCY DISEASE:

Possibly cirrhosis and fatty degeneration of liver, hardening of the arteries, and Alzheimer's disease. (For deficiency symptoms, see section 119.)

BEST NATURAL SOURCES:

Egg yolks, brain, heart, green leafy vegetables, yeast, liver, wheat germ, lecithin (in small amounts).

SUPPLEMENTS:

Six lecithin capsules, made from soybeans, contain 244 mg. each of inositol and choline.

The average B-complex supplement contains approximately 50 mg. of choline and inositol.

Daily doses most often used are 500 to 1,000 mg.

TOXICITY:

None known.
(See section 277, "Cautions.")

ENEMIES:

Water, sulfa drugs, estrogen, food processing, alcohol.
(See section 239.)

PERSONAL ADVICE:

Always take choline with your other B vitamins.

If you are often nervous or "twitchy," it might help to increase your choline.

If you are taking lecithin, you probably need a chelated calcium supplement to keep your phosphorus and calcium in balance, since choline seems to increase the body's phosphorus.

Try getting more choline into your diet as a way to a better memory.

If you're a heavy drinker, make sure you're giving your liver the choline it needs to do the extra work.

38. Vitamin D (Calciferol, Viosterol, Ergosterol, "Sunshine Vitamin")

FACTS:

Fat soluble. Acquired through sunlight or diet. (Ultraviolet sunrays act on the oils of the skin to produce the vitamin, which is then absorbed into the body.)

When taken orally, vitamin D is absorbed with fats through the intestinal walls.

Measured in international units (IU), or micrograms of cholecalciferol (mcg.).

The RDA for adults is 400 IU, or 5–10 mcg.

Smog reduces the vitamin-D-producing sunshine rays.

After a suntan is established, vitamin-D production through the skin stops.

WHAT IT CAN DO FOR YOU:

Properly utilize calcium and phosphorus necessary for strong bones and teeth.

Taken with vitamins A and C it can aid in preventing colds.

Help in treatment of conjunctivitis.

Aid in assimilating vitamin A.

DEFICIENCY DISEASE:

Rickets, severe tooth decay, osteomalacia, senile osteoporosis. (For deficiency symptoms, see section 119.)

BEST NATURAL SOURCES:

Fish liver oils, sardines, herring, salmon, tuna, milk and dairy products.

SUPPLEMENTS:

Usually supplied in 500 IU capsules, the vitamin itself derived from fish liver oil.

Daily doses most often taken are 400 to 1,000 IU.

TOXICITY:

A dosage of 25,000 IU daily over an extended period of time can produce toxic effects in adults.

Dosages of over 5,000 IU daily might affect some individuals adversely.

Signs of toxicity are unusual thirst, sore eyes, itching skin, vomiting, diarrhea, urinary urgency, and abnormal calcium deposits in blood vessel walls, liver, lungs, kidney, and stomach.

(See section 277, "Cautions.")

ENEMIES:

Mineral oil, smog. (See section 239.)

PERSONAL ADVICE:

City dwellers, especially those in areas of high smog density, should increase their vitamin D intake.

Night workers, nuns, and others whose clothing or life-style keeps them from sunlight should increase the D in their diet.

If you're taking an anticonvulsant drug, you most probably need to increase your vitamin D intake.

Children who don't drink D-fortified milk should increase their intake of D.

Dark-skinned people living in northern climates usually need an increase in vitamin D.

Do not supplement your dog's or cat's diet with vitamin D unless your vet specifically advises it.

Vitamin D works best with vitamin A, vitamin C, choline, calcium, and phosphorus.

39. Vitamin E (Tocopherol)

FACTS:

Fat soluble and stored in the liver, fatty tissues, heart, muscles, testes, uterus, blood, and adrenal and pituitary glands.

Formerly measured by weight, but now generally designated according to its biological activity in international units (IU). With this vitamin 1 IU is the same as 1 mg.

Composed of compounds called tocopherols. Of the eight tocopherols—alpha, beta, gamma, delta, epsilon, zeta, eta, and theta—alpha-tocopherol is the most effective.

An active antioxidant, prevents oxidation of fat compounds as well as that of vitamin A, seleniun, two sulfur amino acids, and some vitamin C.

Enhances activity of vitamin A.

The RDA for adults is 8 to 10 IU. (This requirement is based on the National Research Council's 1980 revised allowances.)

From 60 to 70 percent of daily doses are excreted in feces. Unlike other fat-soluble vitamins, E is stored in the body for a relatively short time, much like B and C.

Important as a vasodilator and an anticoagulant.

Products with 25 mcg. of selenium for each 200 units of E increase E's potency.

WHAT IT CAN DO FOR YOU:

Keep you looking younger by retarding cellular aging due to oxidation.

Supply oxygen to the body to give you more endurance.

Protect your lungs against air pollution by working with vitamin A.

Prevent and dissolve blood clots.

Alleviate fatigue.

Prevent thick scar formation externally (when applied topically—it can be absorbed through the skin) and internally.

Accelerate healing of burns.

Working as a diuretic, it can lower blood pressure.

Aid in prevention of miscarriages.

Help alleviate leg cramps and "charley horse."

DEFICIENCY DISEASE:

Destruction of red blood cells, muscle degeneration, some anemias, and productive disorders. (For deficiency symptoms, see section 119.)

BEST NATURAL SOURCES:

Wheat germ, soybeans, vegetable oils, broccoli, Brussels sprouts, leafy greens, spinach, enriched flour, whole wheat, whole-grain cereals, eggs.

SUPPLEMENTS:

Available in oil-base capsules as well as water-dispersible dry tablets.

Usually supplied in strengths from 100 to 1,000 IU. The dry form is recommended for anyone who cannot tolerate oil or whose skin condition is aggravated by oil (also best for people over forty).

Daily doses most often used are 200 to 1,200 IU.

TOXICITY:

Essentially nontoxic.
(See section 277, "Cautions.")

ENEMIES:

Heat, oxygen, freezing temperatures, food processing, iron, chlorine, mineral oil. (See section 239.)

PERSONAL ADVICE:

If you're on a diet high in polyunsaturated oils, you might need additional vitamin E.

Inorganic iron (ferrous sulfate) destroys vitamin E, so the two should not be taken together. If you're using a supplement containing any ferrous sulfate, E should be taken at least eight hours before or after.

Ferrous gluconate, peptonate, citrate, or fumarate (organic iron complexes) does not destroy E.

If you have chlorinated drinking water, you need more vitamin E.

Pregnant or lactating women, as well as those on the pill or taking hormones, need increased vitamin E.

I advise women going through menopause to increase their E intake (mixed tocopherols are recommended, 400 to 1,200 IU daily).

40. Vitamin F (Unsaturated Fatty Acids— Linoleic, Linolenic, and Arachidonic)

FACTS:

Fat soluble, made up of unsaturated fatty acids obtained from foods.

Measured in milligrams (mg.).

No RDA has been established, but the National Research Council has suggested that at least one percent of total calories should include essential unsaturated fatty acids.

Unsaturated fat helps burn saturated fat, with intake balanced two to one.

Twelve teaspoons sunflower seeds or eighteen pecan halves can furnish a day's complete supply.

If there is sufficient linoleic acid, the other two fatty acids can be synthesized.

Heavy carbohydrate consumption increases need.

WHAT IT CAN DO FOR YOU:

Aid in preventing cholesterol deposits in the arteries.

Promote healthy skin and hair.

Give some degree of protection against the harmful effects of X rays.

Aid in growth and well-being by influencing glandular activity and making calcium available to cells.

Combat heart disease.

Aid in weight reduction by burning saturated fats.

DEFICIENCY DISEASE:

Eczema, acne. (For deficiency symptoms, see section 119.)

BEST NATURAL SOURCES:

Vegetable oils—wheat germ, linseed, sunflower, safflower, soybean, and peanut—peanuts, sunflower seeds, walnuts, pecans, almonds, avocados.

SUPPLEMENTS:

Comes in capsules of 100- to 150-mg. strengths.

TOXICITY:

No known toxic effects, but an excess can lead to unwanted pounds.
(See section 277, "Cautions.")

ENEMIES:

Saturated fats, heat, oxygen.

PERSONAL ADVICE:

For best absorption of vitamin F, take vitamin E with it at mealtimes.
If you are a heavy carbohydrate consumer, you need more vitamin F.
Anyone worried about cholesterol buildup should be getting the proper intake of F.

Though most nuts are fine sources of unsaturated fatty acids, Brazil nuts and cashews are *not*.

Watch out for fad diets high in saturated fats.

41. Folic Acid (Folacin)

FACTS:

Water soluble, another member of the B complex, also known as B_c or vitamin M.

Measured in micrograms (mcg.).

Essential to the formation of red blood cells.

Aids in protein metabolism.

The official Recommended Daily Allowance for adults is 400 mcg., twice that amount for pregnant women, and 500 mcg. for nursing mothers.

Important for the production of nucleic acids (RNA and DNA).

Essential for division of body cells.

Needed for utilization of sugar and amino acids.

Can be destroyed by being stored, unprotected, at room temperature for extended time periods.

WHAT IT CAN DO FOR YOU:

Improve lactation.

Protect against intestinal parasites and food poisoning.

Promote healthier-looking skin.

Act as an analgesic for pain.

May delay hair graying when used in conjunction with pantothenic acid and PABA.

Increase appetite, if you are debilitated (run down).

Act as a preventive for canker sores.

Help ward off anemia.

DEFICIENCY DISEASE:

Nutritional macrocytic anemia. (For deficiency symptoms, see section 119.)

BEST NATURAL SOURCES:

Deep green leafy vegetables, carrots, tortula yeast, liver, egg yolk, cantaloupe, apricots, pumpkins, avocados, beans, whole wheat and dark rye flour.

SUPPLEMENTS:

Usually supplied in 400-mcg. and 800-mcg. strengths. Strengths of 1 mg. (1,000 mcg.) are available by prescription only.

Dosages of 400 mcg. are sometimes supplied in B-complex formulas, but often only 100 mcg. (check labels).

Daily doses most often used are 400 mcg. to 5 mg.

TOXICITY:

No known toxic effects, though a few people experience allergic skin reactions.

(See section 277, "Cautions.")

ENEMIES:

Water, sulfa drugs, sunlight, estrogen, food processing (especially boiling), heat. (See section 239.)

PERSONAL ADVICE:

If you are a heavy drinker, it is advisable to increase your folic-acid intake.

High vitamin-C intake increases excretion of folic acid, and anyone taking more than 2 g. of C should probably also take more folic acid.

If you are on Dilantin or take estrogens, sulfonamides, phenobarbital, or aspirin, I suggest increasing folic acid.

I've found that many people taking 1 to 5 mg. daily, for a short period of time, have reversed several types of skin discoloration. If this is a problem to you, it's worth checking out a nutritionally oriented doctor about the possibility.

If you are getting sick, or fighting an illness, make sure your stress supplement has ample folic acid. When folic acid is deficient, so are your antibodies.

42. Inositol

FACTS:

Water soluble, another member of the B complex, and a lipotropic.

Measured in milligrams (mg.)

Combines with choline to form lecithin.

Metabolizes fats and cholesterol.

Daily dietary allowances have not yet been established, but the average healthy adult gets approximately 1 g. a day.

Like choline, it has been found important in nourishing brain cells.

WHAT IT CAN DO FOR YOU:

Help lower cholesterol levels.
Promote healthy hair—aid in preventing fallout.
Help in preventing eczema.
Aid in redistribution of body fat.
Produce a calming effect.

DEFICIENCY DISEASE:

Eczema. (For deficiency symptoms, see section 119.)

BEST NATURAL SOURCES:

Liver, brewer's yeast, dried lima beans, beef brains and heart, cantaloupe, grapefruit, raisins, wheat germ, unrefined molasses, peanuts, cabbage.

SUPPLEMENTS:

As with choline, six soybean-based lecithin capsules contain approximately 244 mg. each of inositol and choline.
Available in lecithin powders that mix well with liquids. Most B-complex supplements contain approximately 100 mg. of choline and inositol.
Daily doses most often used are 250 to 500 mg.

TOXICITY:

No known toxic effects.
(See section 277, "Cautions.")

ENEMIES:

Water, sulfa drugs, estrogen, food processing, alcohol, coffee. (See section 239.)

PERSONAL ADVICE:

Take inositol with choline and your other B vitamins.

If you are a heavy coffee drinker, you probably need supplemental inositol.

If you take lecithin, I advise a supplement of chelated calcium to keep your phosphorus and calcium in balance, as both inositol and choline seem to raise phosphorus levels.

A good way to maximize the effectiveness of your vitamin E is to get enough inositol and choline.

43. Vitamin K (Menadione)

FACTS:

Fat soluble.

Usually measured in micrograms (mcg.).

There is a trio of K vitamins. K_1 and K_2 can be formed by natural bacteria in the intestines. K_3 is a synthetic.

No dietary allowance has yet been established, but an adult intake of approximately 300 mcg. is generally considered adequate. Newborn infants need more.

Essential in the formation of prothrombin, a blood-clotting chemical.

WHAT IT CAN DO FOR YOU:

Help in preventing internal bleeding and hemorrhages.
Aid in reducing excessive menstrual flow.
Promote proper blood clotting.

DEFICIENCY DISEASE:

Celiac disease, sprue, colitis. (For deficiency symptoms, see section 119.)

BEST NATURAL SOURCES:

Yogurt, alfalfa, egg yolk, safflower oil, soybean oil, fish liver oils, kelp, leafy green vegetables.

SUPPLEMENTS:

Available in 100 mcg. tablets (though the abundance of natural vitamin K generally makes supplementation unnecessary).
It is not included ordinarily in multiple vitamins.

TOXICITY:

More than 500 mcg. of synthetic vitamin K is not recommended.
(See section 277, "Cautions.")

ENEMIES:

X rays and radiation, frozen foods, aspirin, air pollution, mineral oil. (See section 239.)

PERSONAL ADVICE:

Excessive diarrhea can be a symptom of vitamin K deficiency, but before self-supplementing, see a doctor.

Yogurt is your best defense against a vitamin K deficiency.

If you have nosebleeds often, try increasing your K through natural food sources. Alfalfa tablets might help.

If you are taking an anticoagulant (blood thinner), be aware that this vitamin (even in natural foods) can reverse the drug's effect.

44. Niacin (Nicotinic Acid, Niacinamide, Nicotinamide)

FACTS:

Water soluble and a member of the B-complex family, known as B_3.

Usually measured in milligrams (mg.).

Using the amino acid tryptophan, the body can manufacture its own niacin.

A person whose body is deficient in B_1, B_2, and B_6 will not be able to produce niacin from tryptophan.

Lack of niacin can bring about negative personality changes.

The RDA, according to the National Research Council, is 13 to 19 mg. for adults.

Essential for synthesis of sex hormones (estrogen, progesterone, testosterone), as well as cortisone, throxine, and insulin.

Necessary for healthy nervous system and brain function.

Niacinamide is more generally used since it minimizes the flushing and itching of the skin that frequently occur with the nicotinic acid form of niacin. (The flush, by the way, is not serious and usually disappears in about twenty minutes. Drinking a glass of water helps.)

WHAT IT CAN DO FOR YOU:

Aid in promoting a healthy digestive system, alleviate gastrointestinal disturbances.

Give you healthier-looking skin.

Help prevent and ease severity of migraine headaches.

Increase circulation and reduce high blood pressure.

Ease some attacks of diarrhea.

Reduce the unpleasant symptoms of vertigo in Ménière's syndrome.

Increase energy through proper utilization of food.

Help eliminate canker sores and, often, bad breath.

Reduce cholesterol and triglycerides.

DEFICIENCY DISEASE:

Pellagra. (For deficiency symptoms, see section 119.)

BEST NATURAL SOURCES:

Liver, lean meat, whole-wheat products, brewer's yeast, kidney, wheat germ, fish, eggs, roasted peanuts, the white meat of poultry, avocados, dates, figs, prunes.

SUPPLEMENTS:

Available as niacin and niacinamide. (The only difference is that niacin—nicotinic acid—might cause flushing and niacinamide—nicotinamide—will not. If you prefer niacin, you can minimize the flushing by taking your pill on a full stomach or with an equivalent amount of inositol.)

Usually found in 50- to 1,000-mg. doses in pill and powder form.

Dosages of 50 to 100 mg. are ordinarily included in the better B-complex formulas and multivitamin preparations (check labels).

TOXICITY:

Essentially nontoxic, except for side effects resulting from doses above 100 mg.

Some sensitive individuals might evidence burning or itching skin.

Do not give to animals, especially dogs. It can cause flushing and sweating and great discomfort for the animal.

(See section 277, "Cautions.")

ENEMIES:

Water, sulfa drugs, alcohol, food-processing techniques, sleeping pills, estrogen. (See section 239.)

PERSONAL ADVICE:

If you're taking antibiotics and suddenly find your niacin flushes becoming severe, don't be alarmed. It's quite common. You'll probably be more comfortable if you switch to niacinamide.

If you have a cholesterol problem, increasing your niacin intake can help.

Skin that is particularly sensitive to sunlight is often an early indicator of niacin deficiency.

45. Vitamin P (C Complex, Citrus Bioflavonoids, Rutin, Hesperidin)

FACTS:

Water soluble and composed of citrin, rutin, and hesperidin, as well as flavones and flavonols.

Usually measured in milligrams (mg.).

Necessary for the proper function and absorption of vitamin C.

Flavonoids are the substances that provide that yellow and orange color in citrus foods.

Also called the capillary permeability factor. (P stands for permeability.) The prime function of bioflavonoids is to increase capillary strength and regulate absorption.

Aids vitamin C in keeping connective tissues healthy.

No daily allowance has been established, but most nutritionists agree that for every 500 mg. of vitamin C you should have at least 100 mg. of bioflavonoids.

Works synergistically with vitamin C.

WHAT IT CAN DO FOR YOU:

Prevent vitamin C from being destroyed by oxidation.

Strengthen the walls of capillaries, thereby preventing bruising.

Help build resistance to infection.

Aid in preventing and healing bleeding gums.

Increase the effectiveness of vitamin C.

Help in the treatment of edema and dizziness due to disease of the inner ear.

DEFICIENCY DISEASE:

Capillary fragility. (For deficiency symptoms, see section 119.)

BEST NATURAL SOURCES:

The white skin and segment part of citrus fruit—lemons, oranges, grapefruit. Also in apricots, buckwheat, blackberries, cherries, rose hips.

SUPPLEMENTS:

Available usually in a C complex or by itself. Most often there are 500 mg. of bioflavonoids to 50 mg. of rutin and hesperidin. (If the ratio of rutin and hesperidin is not equal, it should be twice as much rutin.)

All C supplements work better with bioflavonoids.

Most common doses of rutin and hesperidin are 100 mg. three times a day.

TOXICITY:

No known toxicity.
(See section 277, "Cautions.")

ENEMIES:

Water, cooking, heat, light, oxygen, smoking. (See section 239.)

PERSONAL ADVICE:

Menopausal women can usually find some effective relief from hot flashes with an increase in bioflavonoids taken in conjunction with vitamin C.

If your gums bleed frequently when you brush your teeth, make sure you're getting enough rutin and hesperidin.

Anyone with a tendency to bruise easily will benefit from a C supplement with bioflavonoids, rutin, and hesperidin.

46. PABA (Para-aminobenzoic Acid)

FACTS:

Water soluble, one of the newer members of the B-complex family.

Usually measured in milligrams (mg.).

Can be synthesized in the body.

No RDA has yet been established.

Helps form folic acid and is important in the utilization of protein.

Has important sun-screening properties.

Helps in the assimilation—and therefore the effectiveness—of pantothenic acid.

In experiments with animals, it has worked with pantothenic acid to restore gray hair to its natural color.

WHAT IT CAN DO FOR YOU:

Used as an ointment it can protect against sunburn.

Reduce the pain of burns.

Keep skin healthy and smooth.

Help in delaying wrinkles.

Help to restore natural color to your hair.

DEFICIENCY DISEASE:

Eczema. (For deficiency symptoms, see section 119.)

Best Natural Sources:

Liver, brewer's yeast, kidney, whole grains, rice, bran, wheat germ, molasses.

Supplements:

Dosages of 30 to 100 mgs. are often included in good B-complex capsules as well as in high-quality multivitamins.

Available in 30- to 1,000-mg. strengths in regular and time-release form.

Doses most often used are 30 to 100 mg. three times a day.

Toxicity:

No known toxic effects, but long-term programs of high dosages are not recommended.

Symptoms that might indicate an oversupply of PABA are usually nausea and vomiting.

(See section 277, "Cautions.")

Enemies:

Water, sulfa drugs, food-processing techniques, alcohol, estrogen. (See section 239.)

Personal Advice:

Some people claim that the combination of folic acid and PABA has returned their graying hair to its natural color. It has worked on animals, so it is certainly worth a try for anyone looking for an alternative to hair dye.

For this purpose, 1,000 mg. (time release) daily for six days a week is a viable regimen.

If you tend to burn easily in the sun, use PABA as a protective ointment.

Many Hollywood celebrities I know use PABA to prevent wrinkles. It doesn't eliminate them, but it certainly seems to keep them at bay for some people.

If you are taking penicillin, or any sulfa drug, your PABA intake should be increased through natural foods or supplements.

47. Vitamin T

There is very little known about this vitamin, except that it helps in blood coagulation and the forming of platelets. Because of these attributes it is important in warding off certain forms of anemia and hemophilia. No RDA has been established. It is found in sesame seeds and egg yolks, and there is no known toxicity.

48. Vitamin U

Even less is known about vitamin U than vitamin T. It is reputed to play an important role in healing ulcers, but medical opinions vary on this. It is found in raw cabbage and no known toxicity exists.

49. Any Questions About Chapter III?

I live in Los Angeles and hear a lot about environmental pollution. I also hear a lot about how I need to take antioxidants. Could you tell me what antioxidants are and if I really need them?

You really need them. Let me begin by saying that if you live in *any* major urban area today, you're breathing polluted air. Every year 200 million tons of potentially dangerous pollutants are released into the atmosphere.

With each breath you subject your lungs and body to a wide range of pollutants, and no part of you is immune. Antioxidants—vitamins A, C, E, and selenium—are nutrients that are capable of protecting other substances from oxidation. In other words, the free radicals (uncontrolled oxidations that damage cells) that are formed when we inhale pollutants are kept in check by antioxidants.

Vitamin A protects mucous membranes of mouth, nose, throat, and lungs. It also helps protect vitamin C from oxidation, which allows your C to work better.

Vitamin C fights bacterial infections and reduces the effects of allergy-producing substances. It also protects vitamins A, E, and some of the B complex from oxidation.

Vitamin E protects vitamins B and C from oxidation. It has the ability to unite with oxygen and prevent it from being converted into toxic peroxides. It acts as an antipollutant for the lungs.

Selenium and vitamin E must both be present to correct a deficiency in either. The levels of selenium in the blood of people in various cities have been found to bear a direct relationship to cancer mortality. The higher the levels of selenium, the lower the cancer death rate—and vice versa.

I've read that diets high in broccoli, brussels sprouts, and carrots can help reduce the risk of cancer, but I just hate these vegetables. What vitamins can I take instead?

You can get concentrated forms of cruciferous (cabbage, broccoli, brussels sprouts, cauliflower) and carotene-rich (spinach and carrots) vegetables in tablet form. I'd advise taking these supplements daily. Since they are made from vegetables that are picked ripe, carefully washed, and quickly dehydrated without cooking—as well as being fortified with vitamins A, C, and E, beta-carotene, and selenium—they'll provide you with optimal nutritional value.

Can you tell me how choline is helpful in the treatment of Alzheimer's disease?

Alzheimer's disease, which is a slow loss of mental faculties, and becoming so common among older individuals that many doctors are referring to it as "the disease of the eighties," seems to be caused by a depletion in central nervous system reserves of the neurotransmitter acetylcholine (not by a virus or aluminum, as previously suspected).

It has been found that patients with Alzheimer's syndrome are not only deficient in acetylcholine, but also lack the enzyme that catalyzes its production—choline acetyltransferase. Ingestion of more choline can apparently prevent existing acetylcholine from being broken down.

There is still no specific treatment for the disease, but it's been found that certain medications might worsen a patient's condition (for example, hypnotics such as flurazepam [Dalmane], drugs for heart disease, and those given for intestinal cramping).

IV

Your Mineral Essentials

50. Calcium

FACTS:

There is more calcium in the body than any other mineral.

Calcium and phosphorus work together for healthy bones and teeth.

Calcium and magnesium work together for cardiovascular health.

Almost all of the body's calcium (two to three pounds) is found in the bones and teeth.

Twenty percent of an adult's bone calcium is reabsorbed and replaced every year. (New bone cells form as old ones break down.)

Calcium must exist in a two-to-one relationship with phosphorus (two parts calcium to one part phosphorus).

In order for calcium to be absorbed, the body must have sufficient vitamin D.

For adults, 800 to 1,200 mg. is the RDA.

Calcium and iron are the two minerals most deficient in the American woman's diet.

WHAT IT CAN DO FOR YOU:

Maintain strong bones and healthy teeth.
Keep your heart beating regularly.
Alleviate insomnia.
Help metabolize your body's iron.
Aid your nervous system, especially in impulse transmission.

DEFICIENCY DISEASE:

Rickets, osteomalacia, osteoporosis—commonly known as brittle bones. (See section 119 for symptoms.)

BEST NATURAL SOURCES:

Milk and milk products, all cheeses, soybeans, sardines, salmon, peanuts, walnuts, sunflower seeds, dried beans, green vegetables.

SUPPLEMENTS:

Most often available in 100- to 500-mg. tablets.
Bonemeal is a fairly common supplement and a good source of the mineral, though some people find calcium gluconate (a vegetarian source) or calcium lactate (a milk sugar derivative) easier to absorb. (Gluconate is more potent than lactate.)
The best form is chelated calcium tablets.
Many good multivitamin and multimineral preparations include calcium.
When combined with magnesium, the ratio should be twice as much calcium as magnesium. Dolomite is a natural form of calcium and magnesium, and no vitamin

D is needed for assimilation. Five dolomite tablets are equivalent to 750 mg. of calcium.

Doses most often used are 800 to 2,000 mg. per day.

Both bonemeal (calcium and phosphorus) and dolomite can have high lead contents; check with the manufacturer for an analysis.

TOXICITY:

Excessive daily intake of over 2,000 mg. might lead to hypercalcemia.

(See section 277, "Cautions.")

ENEMIES:

Large quantities of fat, oxalic acid (found in chocolate and rhubarb), and phytic acid (found in grains) are capable of preventing proper calcium absorption.

PERSONAL ADVICE:

If you are afflicted with backaches, dolomite, chelated calcium, or bonemeal supplements might help.

Menstrual-cramp sufferers can often find relief by increasing their calcium intake.

Teenagers who suffer from "growing pains" will usually find that they disappear with an increase in calcium consumption.

Hypoglycemics could use more calcium. (I recommend chelated calcium, for best absorption, in doses of 1,000 to 1,500 mg. daily.)

Calcium works best with vitamins A, C, D; iron, magnesium, and phosphorus. (Too much phosphorus, though, can deplete calcium.)

51. Chlorine

FACTS:

Regulates the blood's alkaline-acid balance.
Works with sodium and potassium in a compound form.
Aids in the cleaning of body wastes by helping the liver to function.
No dietary allowance has been established, but if your daily salt intake is average, you are getting enough.

WHAT IT CAN DO FOR YOU:

Aid in digestion.
Help keep you limber.

DEFICIENCY DISEASE:

Loss of hair and teeth.

BEST NATURAL SOURCES:

Table salt, kelp, olives.

SUPPLEMENTS:

Most good multimineral preparations include it.

TOXICITY:

Over 15 g. can cause unpleasant side effects.
(See section 277, "Cautions.")

PERSONAL ADVICE:

If you have chlorine in your drinking water, you aren't getting all the vitamin E you think. (Chlorinated water destroys vitamin E.)

Anyone who drinks chlorinated water would be well advised to eat yogurt—a good way to replace the intestinal bacteria the chlorine destroys.

52. Chromium

FACTS:

Works with insulin in the metabolism of sugar.

Helps bring protein to where it's needed.

No official dietary allowance has been established, but 50 to 200 mcg. is an average adult intake.

As you get older, you retain less chromium in your body.

WHAT IT CAN DO FOR YOU:

Aid growth.

Help prevent and lower high blood pressure.

Work as a deterrent for diabetes.

DEFICIENCY DISEASE:

A suspected factor in arteriosclerosis and diabetes.

BEST NATURAL SOURCES:

Meat, shellfish, chicken, corn oil, clams, brewer's yeast.

SUPPLEMENTS:

May be found in the better multimineral preparations.
(Glucose tolerance factor is the preferred form.)

TOXICITY:

No known toxicity.
(See section 277, "Cautions.")

PERSONAL ADVICE:

If you are low in chromium (a hair analysis might
show this—see section 118), you could try a zinc
supplement. For some reason, chelated zinc seems to
substitute well for deficient chromium.

53. Cobalt

FACTS:

A mineral that is part of vitamin B_{12}.
Usually measured in micrograms (mcg.).
Essential for red blood cells.
Must be obtained from food sources.
No daily allowance has been set for this mineral, and
only very small amounts are necessary in the diet
(usually no more than 8 mcg.).

WHAT IT CAN DO FOR YOU:

Stave off anemia.

DEFICIENCY DISEASE:

Anemia.

BEST NATURAL SOURCES:

Meat, kidney, liver, milk, oysters, clams.

SUPPLEMENTS:

Rarely found in supplement form.

TOXICITY:

No known toxicity.
(See section 277, "Cautions.")

ENEMIES:

Whatever is antagonistic to B_{12}.

PERSONAL ADVICE:

If you're a strict vegetarian, you are much more likely to be deficient in this mineral than someone who includes meat and shellfish in his or her diet.

54. Copper

FACTS:

Required to convert the body's iron into hemoglobin.
Can reach the bloodstream fifteen minutes after ingestion.
Makes the amino acid tyrosine usable, allowing it to work as the pigmenting factor for hair and skin.
Present in cigarettes, birth-control pills, and automobile pollution.
Essential for the utilization of vitamin C.

The RDA has not been set by the National Research Council, but 2 to 3 mg. for adults is suggested.

What It Can Do For You:

Keep your energy up by aiding in effective iron absorption.

Deficiency Disease:

Anemia, edema.

Natural Food Sources:

Dried beans, peas, whole wheat, prunes, calf and beef liver, shrimp, most seafood.

Supplements:

Usually available in multivitamin and multimineral supplements in 2-mg. doses.

Toxicity:

Rare.
(See section 277, "Cautions.")

Enemies:

Not easily destroyed.

Personal Advice:

As essential as copper is, I rarely suggest special supplementation. An excess seems to lower zinc level and produces insomnia, hair loss, irregular menses, and depression.

If you eat enough whole-grain products and fresh green leafy vegetables, as well as liver, you don't have to worry about your copper intake.

55. Fluorine

FACTS:

Part of the synthetic compound sodium fluoride (the type added to drinking water) and calcium fluoride (a natural substance).

Decreases chances of dental caries, though too much can discolor teeth.

No RDA has been established, but most people get about 1 mg. daily from fluoridated drinking water. (Dosages of 1.5 to 4 mg. are suggested by the National Academy of Sciences–National Research Council.)

WHAT IT CAN DO FOR YOU:

Reduce tooth decay.
Strengthen bones.

DEFICIENCY DISEASE:

Tooth decay.

BEST NATURAL SOURCES:

Fluoridated drinking water, seafood, gelatin.

SUPPLEMENTS:

Not ordinarily found in multimineral supplements.
Available in prescription multivitamins for children in areas without fluoridated water.

TOXICITY:

Dosages of 20 to 80 mg. per day can produce toxic effects.
(See section 277, "Cautions.")

ENEMIES:

Aluminum salts of fluorine.

PERSONAL ADVICE:

Don't take additional fluoride unless it is prescribed by a physician or dentist.

56. Iodine (Iodide)

FACTS:

Two-thirds of the body's iodine is in the thyroid gland.
Since the thyroid gland controls metabolism, and iodine influences the thyroid, an undersupply of this mineral can result in slow mental reaction, weight gain, and lack of energy.
The RDA, as established by the National Research Council, is 150 mcg. for adults (1 mcg. per kilogram of body weight) and 175 to 200 mcg. for pregnant and lactating women respectively.

WHAT IT CAN DO FOR YOU:

Help you with dieting by burning excess fat.
Promote proper growth.
Give you more energy.
Improve mental alacrity.
Promote healthy hair, nails, skin, and teeth.

DEFICIENCY DISEASE:

Goiter, hypothyroidism.

BEST NATURAL SOURCES:

Kelp, vegetables grown in iodine-rich soil, onions, all seafood.

SUPPLEMENTS:

Available in multimineral and high-potency vitamin supplements in doses of 0.15 mg.
Natural kelp is a good source of supplemental iodine.

TOXICITY:

No known toxicity from natural iodine, though iodine as a drug can be harmful if prescribed incorrectly.
(See section 277, "Cautions.")

ENEMIES:

Food processing, nutrient-poor soil.

PERSONAL ADVICE:

Aside from kelp, and the iodine included in multimineral and multivitamin preparations, I don't recommend additional supplements unless you're advised by a doctor to take them.

If you use salt and live in the Midwest, where iodine-poor soil is common, make sure the salt is iodized.

If you are inclined to eat excessive amounts of raw cabbage, you might *not* be getting the iodine you need, because there are elements in the cabbage that prevent proper utilization of the iodine. This being the case, you should consider a kelp supplement.

57. Iron

FACTS:

Essential and required for life, necessary for the production of hemoglobin (red blood corpuscles), myoglobin (red pigment in muscles), and certain enzymes.

Iron and calcium are the two major dietary deficiencies of American women.

Only about 8 percent of your total iron intake is absorbed and actually enters your bloodstream.

An average 150-pound adult has about 4 g. of iron in his or her body. Hemoglobin, which accounts for most of the iron, is recycled and reutilized as blood cells are replaced every 120 days. Iron bound to protein (ferritin) is stored in the body, as is tissue iron (present in myoglobin) in very small amounts.

The RDA, according to the National Research Council, is 10 to 18 mg. for adults, and 30 to 60 mg. for pregnant and lactating women.

In one month, women lose almost twice as much iron as men.

Copper, cobalt, manganese, and vitamin C are necessary to assimilate iron.

Iron is necessary for proper metabolization of B vitamins.

WHAT IT CAN DO FOR YOU:

Aid growth.
Promote resistance to disease.
Prevent fatigue.
Cure and prevent iron-deficiency anemia.
Bring back good skin tone.

DEFICIENCY DISEASE:

Iron-deficiency anemia. (For deficiency symptoms, see section 119.)

BEST NATURAL SOURCES:

Pork liver; beef kidney, heart, and liver; farina, raw clams, dried peaches, red meat, egg yolks, oysters, nuts, beans, asparagus, molasses, oatmeal.

SUPPLEMENTS:

The most assimilable form of iron is hydrolyzed-protein chelate, which means organic iron that has been processed for fastest assimilation. This form is nonconstipating and easy on sensitive systems.

Ferrous sulfate, inorganic iron, appears in many vitamin and mineral supplements and can destroy vitamin E (they should be taken at least eight hours apart). Check labels; many drugstore formulas contain ferrous sulfate.

Supplements with organic iron—ferrous gluconate, ferrous fumarate, ferrous citrate, or ferrous peptonate— do not neutralize vitamin E. They are available in a wide variety of doses, usually up to 320 mg.

TOXICITY:

Rare in healthy, normal individuals. Excessive doses, though, can be a hazard for children. (See section 277, "Cautions.") Should not be taken by anyone with sickle-cell anemia, hemochromotosis, or thalassemia.

ENEMIES:

Phosphoproteins in eggs and phytates in unleavened whole wheat reduce iron availability to the body.

PERSONAL ADVICE:

If you are a woman, I recommend a chelated or hemoglobin iron supplement. Check the label on your multivitamin or multimineral preparation and see what you are already getting, then guide yourself accordingly. (Remember, if the iron in your preparation is ferrous sulfate, you're losing your vitamin E.)

Keep your iron supplements out of the reach of children.

Coffee drinkers, as well as tea drinkers, be aware that if you consume large quantities of either beverage, you are most likely inhibiting your iron absorption.

If you are pregnant, check with your doctor before taking iron or iron-fortified vitamin supplements. (Iron poisoning has been found in children whose mothers have taken too many iron pills during pregnancy.)

58. Magnesium

FACTS:

Necessary for calcium and vitamin-C metabolism, as well as that of phosphorus, sodium, and potassium.
Measured in milligrams (mg.).
Essential for effective nerve and muscle functioning.
Important for converting blood sugar into energy.
Known as the antistress mineral.
Alcoholics are usually deficient.
Adults need 300 to 450 mg. daily, slightly more for pregnant and lactating women, according to the National Research Council.
The human body contains approximately 21 g. of magnesium.

WHAT IT CAN DO FOR YOU:

Aid in fighting depression.
Promote a healthier cardiovascular system and help prevent heart attacks.
Keep teeth healthier.
Help prevent calcium deposits, kidney stones, and gallstones.
Bring relief from indigestion.
Combined with calcium can work as a natural tranquilizer.

DEFICIENCY DISEASE:

(For deficiency symptoms, see section 119.)

Best Natural Sources:

Figs, lemons, grapefruit, yellow corn, almonds, nuts, seeds, dark green vegetables, apples.

Supplements:

Chelated magnesium and calcium in perfect balance (half as much magnesium as calcium) is a fine supplement.

Available in multivitamin and multimineral preparations.

Can be purchased as magnesium oxide (250-mg. strength equals 150 mg. per tablet).

Commonly available in 133.3-mg. strengths and taken four times a day.

Supplements of magnesium should not be taken after meals, since the mineral does neutralize stomach acidity.

Toxicity:

Large amounts, over an extended period of time, can be toxic if your calcium and phosphorus intakes are high.

(See section 277, "Cautions.")

Enemies:

Diuretics, alcohol. (See section 239.)

Personal Advice:

If you are a drinker, I suggest you increase your intake of magnesium.

Women who are on the pill or taking estrogen in any form would be well advised to take larger amounts of magnesium.

If you are a heavy consumer of nuts, seeds, and green vegetables, you probably get ample magnesium—as does anyone who lives in an area with hard water.

Magnesium works best with vitamin A, calcium, and phosphorus.

59. Manganese

FACTS:

Helps activate enzymes necessary for the body's proper use of biotin, B_1, and vitamin C.

Needed for normal bone structure.

Measured in milligrams (mg.).

Important in the formation of thyroxine, the principal hormone of the thyroid gland.

Necessary for the proper digestion and utilization of food.

No official daily allowance has been set, but 2.5 to 5 mg. is generally accepted to be the average adult requirement.

Important for reproduction and normal central nervous system function.

WHAT IT CAN DO FOR YOU:

Help eliminate fatigue.
Aid in muscle reflexes.
Improve memory.
Reduce nervous irritability.

DEFICIENCY DISEASE:

Ataxia.

BEST NATURAL SOURCES:

Nuts, green leafy vegetables, peas, beets, egg yolks, whole-grain cereals.

SUPPLEMENTS:

Most often found in multivitamin and multimineral combinations in dosages of 1 to 9 mg.

TOXICITY:

Rare, except from industrial sources.
(See section 277, "Cautions.")

ENEMIES:

Large intakes of calcium and phosphorus will inhibit absorption.

PERSONAL ADVICE:

If you suffer from recurrent dizziness, you might try adding more manganese to your diet.

I advise absentminded people, or anyone with memory problems, to make sure they are getting enough of this mineral.

Heavy milk drinkers and meat eaters need increased manganese.

60. Molybdenum

FACTS:

Aids in carbohydrate and fat metabolism.

A vital part of the enzyme responsible for iron utilization.

No dietary allowance has been set, but the estimated daily intake of 150 to 500 mcg. has generally been accepted as the adequate human requirement.

WHAT IT CAN DO FOR YOU:

Help in preventing anemia.
Promote general well-being.

DEFICIENCY DISEASE:

None known.

BEST NATURAL SOURCES:

Dark green leafy vegetables, whole grains, legumes.

SUPPLEMENTS:

Not ordinarily available.

TOXICITY:

Rare, but 5 to 10 parts per million has been considered toxic.
(See section 277, "Cautions.")

PERSONAL ADVICE:

As important as molybdenum is, there seems no need for supplementation unless all the food you consume comes from nutrient-deficient soil.

61. Phosphorus

FACTS:

Present in every cell in the body.

Vitamin D and calcium are essential to proper phosphorus functioning.

Calcium and phosphorus should be balanced two to one to work correctly (twice as much calcium as phosphorus).

Involved in virtually all physiological chemical reactions.

Necessary for normal bone and tooth structure.

Niacin cannot be assimilated without phosphorus.

Important for heart regularity.

Essential for normal kidney functioning.

Needed for the transference of nerve impulses.

The RDA is 800 to 1,200 mg. for adults, the higher levels for pregnant and lactating women.

WHAT IT CAN DO FOR YOU:

Aid in growth and body repair.

Provide energy and vigor by helping in the metabolization of fats and starches.

Lessen the pain of arthritis.

Promote healthy gums and teeth.

DEFICIENCY DISEASE:

Rickets, pyorrhea.

BEST NATURAL SOURCES:

Fish, poultry, meat, whole grains, eggs, nuts, seeds.

SUPPLEMENTS:

Bonemeal is a fine natural source of phosphorus. (Make sure vitamin D has been added to help assimilation.)

TOXICITY:

No known toxicity.
(See section 277, "Cautions.")

ENEMIES:

Too much iron, aluminum, and magnesium can render phosphorus ineffective.

PERSONAL ADVICE:

When you get too much phosphorus, you throw off your mineral balance and decrease your calcium. Our diets are usually high in phosphorus—since it does occur in almost every natural food—and therefore calcium deficiencies are frequent. Be aware of this and adjust your diet accordingly.

If you're over forty, you should cut down on your weekly meat consumption and eat more leafy vegetables and drink milk. The reason for this is that after forty our kidneys don't help excrete excess phosphorus, and calcium is again depleted. Be on the lookout for foods preserved with phosphates and consider that as part of your phosphorus intake.

62. Potassium

FACTS:

Works with sodium to regulate the body's water balance and normalize heart rhythms. (Potassium works inside the cells, sodium works just outside them.)

Nerve and muscle functions suffer when the sodium-potassium balance is off.

Hypoglycemia (low blood sugar) causes potassium loss, as does a long fast or severe diarrhea.

No dietary allowance has been set, but 1,875 to 5,625 mg. is considered a healthy daily adult intake.

Both mental and physical stress can lead to a potassium deficiency.

WHAT IT CAN DO FOR YOU:

Aid in clear thinking by sending oxygen to the brain.
Help dispose of body wastes.
Assist in reducing blood pressure.
Aid in allergy treatment.

DEFICIENCY DISEASE:

Edema, hypoglycemia. (For deficiency symptoms, see section 119.)

BEST NATURAL SOURCES:

Citrus fruits, cantaloupe, tomatoes, watercress, all green leafy vegetables, mint leaves, sunflower seeds, bananas, potatoes.

SUPPLEMENTS:

Available in most high-potency multivitamin and multimineral preparations.

Inorganic potassium "salts" are the sulfate (alum), the chloride, the oxide, and the carbonate. Organic potassium refers to the gluconate, the citrate, and the fumarate.

Can be bought separately as potassium gluconate, citrate, or chloride in dosages up to nearly 600 mg. (99 mg. elemental potassium).

TOXICITY:

A dosage of 25 g. of potassium chloride can cause toxicity.

(See section 277, "Cautions.")

ENEMIES:

Alcohol, coffee, sugar, diuretics. (See section 239.)

PERSONAL ADVICE:

If you drink large amounts of coffee, you might find that the fatigue you're fighting is due to the potassium loss you're suffering from.

Heavy drinkers and anyone with a hungry sweet tooth should be aware that their potassium levels are probably low.

If you have low blood sugar, you are likely to be losing potassium while retaining water. And if you take a diuretic, you'll lose even more potassium! Watch your diet, increase your green vegetables, and take enough magnesium to regain your mineral balance.

Losing weight on a low-carbohydrate diet might not be the only thing you're losing. Chances are your potassium level is down. Watch out for weakness and poor reflexes.

63. Selenium

FACTS:

Vitamin E and selenium are synergistic. This means that the two together are stronger than the sum of the equal parts.

Both vitamin E and selenium are antioxidants, preventing or at least slowing down aging and hardening of tissues through oxidation.

Males appear to have a greater need for selenium. Almost half their body's supply concentrates in the testicles and portions of the seminal ducts adjacent to the prostate gland. Also, selenium is lost in the semen.

No official dietary allowance has yet been set for this mineral, but the general dosage is between 50 and 200 mcg. It is not advisable to exceed 200 mcg. daily.

WHAT IT CAN DO FOR YOU:

Aid in keeping youthful elasticity in tissues.
Alleviate hot flashes and menopausal distress.
Help in treatment and prevention of dandruff.
Possibly neutralize certain carcinogens and provide protection from some cancers.

Deficiency Disease:

Premature stamina loss.

Best Natural Sources:

Wheat germ, bran, tuna fish, onions, tomatoes, broccoli.

Supplements:

Available in small microgram doses (25 to 100 mcg. is most often used).

Also available combined with vitamin E and other antioxidants.

Natural foods supply sufficient amounts when eaten regularly.

Toxicity:

Doses above 5 parts per million can be toxic.
(See section 277, "Cautions.")

Enemies:

Food-processing techniques.

Personal Advice:

Selenium was discovered only a little more than twenty years ago. We've just begun to recognize its importance in human nutrition. Until more is known, I advise taking only moderate supplements.

64. Sodium

FACTS:

Sodium and potassium were discovered together and both found to be essential for normal growth.

High intakes of sodium (salt) will result in a depletion of potassium.

Diets high in sodium usually account for many instances of high blood pressure.

There is no official allowance, but a daily single gram of sodium chloride has been suggested for each kilogram of water drunk (or 1,100 to 3,300 mg. daily). Sodium aids in keeping calcium and other minerals in the blood soluble.

WHAT IT CAN DO FOR YOU:

Aid in preventing heat prostration or sunstroke.
Help your nerves and muscles function properly.

DEFICIENCY DISEASE:

Impaired carbohydrate digestion, possibly neuralgia.

BEST NATURAL SOURCES:

Salt, shellfish, carrots, beets, artichokes, dried beef, brains, kidney, bacon.

SUPPLEMENTS:

Rarely needed, but if so, kelp is a safe and nutritive supplement.

TOXICITY:

Over 14 g. of sodium chloride daily can produce toxic effects.

(See section 277, "Cautions.")

PERSONAL ADVICE:

If you think you don't eat much salt, see sections 257 and 258 and think again.

If you have high blood pressure, cut down on your salt intake by reading the labels on the foods you buy. Look for Salt, Sodium Chloride, or the chemical symbol *NaCl*.

Adding sodium to your diet is as easy as a shake of salt, but subtracting it can be difficult. Avoid luncheon meats, frankfurters, salted cured meats such as ham, bacon, corned beef, and condiments—ketchup, chili sauce, soy sauce, mustard. Don't use baking powder or baking soda in cooking.

65. Sulfur

FACTS:

Essential for healthy hair, skin, and nails.

Helps maintain oxygen balance necessary for proper brain function.

Works with B-complex vitamins for basic body metabolism and is part of tissue-building amino acids.

Aids the liver in bile secretion.

No RDA has been set, but a diet sufficient in protein will generally be sufficient in sulfur.

WHAT IT CAN DO FOR YOU:

Tone up skin and make hair more lustrous.
Help fight bacterial infections.

DEFICIENCY DISEASE:

None known.

BEST NATURAL SOURCES:

Lean beef, dried beans, fish, eggs, cabbage.

SUPPLEMENTS:

Not readily available as a food supplement.
Can be found in topical ointments and creams for
skin problems.

TOXICITY:

No known toxicity from organic sulfur, but ill effects
may occur from large amounts of inorganic sulfur.
(See section 277, "Cautions.")

PERSONAL ADVICE:

If you're getting enough protein in your daily meals,
you are, most likely, getting enough sulfur.
Sulfur creams and ointments have been remarkably
successful in treating a variety of skin problems. Check
the ingredients in the preparation you are now using.
There are many fine natural preparations available at
health-food centers.

66. Vanadium

FACTS:

Inhibits the formation of cholesterol in blood vessels. No dietary allowance set.

WHAT IT CAN DO FOR YOU:

Aid in preventing heart attacks.

DEFICIENCY DISEASE:

None known.

BEST NATURAL SOURCES:

Fish.

SUPPLEMENTS:

Not available.

TOXICITY:

Can easily be toxic if taken in synthetic form. (See section 277, "Cautions.")

PERSONAL ADVICE:

This is not one of the minerals that needs to be supplemented. A good fish dinner will supply you with the vanadium you need.

67. Zinc

FACTS:

Zinc acts as a traffic policeman, directing and oversee-ing the efficient flow of body processes, the mainte-nance of enzyme systems and cells.

Essential for protein synthesis.

Governs the contractibility of muscles.

Helps in the formation of insulin.

Important for blood stability and in maintaining the body's acid-alkaline balance.

Exerts a normalizing effect on the prostate and is important in the development of all reproductive organs.

New studies indicate its importance in brain function and the treatment of schizophrenia.

Strong evidence of its requirement for the synthesis of DNA.

The RDA, as set by the National Research Council, is 15 mg. for adults (slightly higher allowances for preg-nant and lactating women).

Excessive sweating can cause a loss of as much as 3 mg. of zinc per day.

Most zinc in foods is lost in processing or never exists in substantial amount due to nutrient-poor soil.

WHAT IT CAN DO FOR YOU:

Accelerate healing time for internal and external wounds.

Get rid of white spots on the fingernails.

Help eliminate loss of taste.

Aid in the treatment of infertility.

Help avoid prostate problems.

Promote growth and mental alertness.

Help decrease cholesterol deposits.
Aid in the treatment of mental disorders.

Deficiency Disease:

Possibly prostatic hypertrophy (noncancerous enlargement of the prostate gland), arteriosclerosis.

Best Natural Sources:

Round steak, lamb chops, pork loin, wheat germ, brewer's yeast, pumpkin seeds, eggs, nonfat dry milk, ground mustard.

Supplements:

Available in all good multivitamin and multimineral preparations.

Can be bought as zinc-sulfate or zinc-gluconate tablets in doses ranging from 15 to over 300 mg. Both zinc sulfate and zinc gluconate seem to be equally effective, but zinc gluconate appears to be more easily tolerated.

Chelated zinc is the best way to take zinc.

Zinc is also available in combination with vitamin C, magnesium, and the B-complex vitamins.

Toxicity:

Virtually nontoxic, except when there is an excessive intake and the food ingested has been stored in galvanized containers. Doses over 150 mg. are not recommended.

(See section 277, "Cautions.")

PERSONAL ADVICE:

You need higher intakes of zinc if you are taking large amounts of vitamin B_6. This is also true if you are an alcoholic or a diabetic.

Men with prostate problems—and without them—would be well advised to keep their zinc levels up.

I have seen success in cases of impotence with a supplement program of B_6 and zinc.

Elderly people concerned about senility might find a zinc and manganese supplement beneficial.

If you are bothered by irregular menses, you might try a zinc supplement before resorting to hormone treatments to establish regularity.

Remember, if you are adding zinc to your diet, you will increase your need for vitamin A. (Zinc works best with vitamin A, calcium, and phosphorus.)

68. Water

FACTS:

The simple truth is that this is our most important nutrient. One-half to three-fourths of the body's weight is water.

A human being can live for weeks without food, but only for a few days without water.

Water is the basic solvent for all the products of digestion.

Essential for removing wastes.

There is no specific dietary allowance, since water loss varies with climate, situations, and individuals, but under ordinary circumstances six glasses daily is considered healthy.

Regulates body temperature.

WHAT IT CAN DO FOR YOU:

Keep all your bodily functions functioning.
Aid in dieting by depressing appetite before meals.
Help prevent constipation.

DEFICIENCY DISEASE:

Dehydration.

BEST NATURAL SOURCES:

Drinking water and juices, eating fruits and vegetables.

SUPPLEMENTS:

All drinkable liquids can substitute for our daily
water requirements.

TOXICITY:

No known toxicity, but an intake of one and a half
gallons (that's sixteen to twenty-four glasses) in about
an hour could be dangerous to an adult. It could kill an
infant.

PERSONAL ADVICE:

I advise six to eight glasses of water daily, to be
drunk a half hour before meals, for anyone who's
dieting.
If you're running a fever, be sure to drink lots of
water to prevent dehydration and to flush the system of
wastes.

If you live in an area where there is hard water, you're probably getting more calcium and magnesium than you think.

69. Any Questions About Chapter IV?

I know that water is good for me, but with all the pollution in rivers and streams these days, how can I tell if my tap water is safe to drink?

The best thing to do if you want to find out if there are contaminants in your water is to contact your local water superintendent and ask for the results of water-sampling tests and sanitary surveys; then ask to see the Public Health Service standards, so that you'll be able to compare the former with the latter. You can also have your water tested for contaminants at most local hospital laboratories.

Bottled water might seem to be the logical alternative if you're concerned, but be aware that some bottled water is just processed tap·water to which minerals, with or without carbonation, have been added. Although most major brands are probably free of organic carcinogens, studies have shown that there are quite a few bottling plants with sanitary deficiencies. It's also wise to check with the bottler about the source of their water and choose one whose source is natural spring water taken from a spring in a nonindustrial area.

V

Protein—And Those Amazing Amino Acids

70. The Protein–Amino Acid Connection

Protein is a life necessity in the diet of man and all animals. Actually, though, it is not protein itself that is required, but the amino acids which are the building blocks of protein.

> If any essential amino acid is low or missing, the effectiveness of all the others will be proportionately reduced.

Amino acids, which combined with nitrogen form thousands of different proteins, are not only the units from which proteins are formed, but are also the end product of protein digestion.

There are twenty-two known amino acids. Eight of these are called *essential amino acids*. These essential amino acids *cannot*, like the others, be manufactured by the human body and *must* be obtained from food or supplements. A ninth amino acid, histidine, is considered essential only for infants and children.

THE 22 AMINO ACIDS
(Essential amino acids are marked with asterisks.)

Alanine
Arginine
Asparagine
Aspartic acid
Cysteine
Cystine
Glutamic acid
Glutamine
Glycine
*Histidine (for infants and children)
*Isoleucine
*Leucine
*Lysine
*Methionine
Ornithine
*Phenylalanine
Proline
Serine
*Threonine
*Tryptophan
Tyrosine
*Valine

In order for the body to effectively use and synthesize protein, all the essential amino acids must be present and in the proper proportions. Even the temporary absence of a single essential amino acid can adversely affect protein synthesis. In fact, whatever essential amino acid is low or missing will proportionately reduce the effectiveness of all the others.

71. How Much Protein Do You Need, Really?

Everyone's protein requirements differ, depending on a variety of factors including health, age, and size. Actually, the larger and younger you are, the more you need. To estimate your own personal daily recommended allowance, see the chart below.

AGE	1–3	4–6	7–10	11–14	15–18	19 and over
POUND KEY	0.82	0.68	0.55	0.45	0.40	0.36

- Find the pound key under your age group.
- Multiply that number by your weight.
- The result will be your daily protein requirement in grams.

    Example: You weigh 100 pounds and are 33 years old. Your pound key is 0.36.

    0.36 × 100 = 36 g.—your daily protein requirement.

An average minimum protein requirement is around 45 g. a day. That's 15 g. or about half an ounce per meal. Make sure you get enough at breakfast.

72. Types of Protein—What's the Difference?

All proteins are not the same, though they're manufactured from the same twenty-two amino acids. They have different functions and work in different areas of the body.

There are basically two types of protein—complete protein and incomplete protein.

Complete protein provides the proper balance of eight necessary amino acids that build tissues and is found in foods of animal origin such as meats, poultry, seafood, eggs, milk, and cheese.

Incomplete protein lacks certain essential amino acids and is not used efficiently when eaten alone. However, when combined with small amounts of animal-source protein, it becomes complete. It is found in seeds, nuts, peas, grains, and beans.

Mixing complete and incomplete proteins can give you better nutrition than having either one alone. A good rice-and-beans dish with some cheese can be just as nourishing, less expensive, and lower in fat than a steak.

73. Protein Myths

A lot of people seem to think that protein is nonfattening. This misconception has frustrated many a determined dieter who forgoes bread but eats healthy portions of steak and wonders where the weight is coming from. The fact is

- 1 g. protein = 4 calories
- 1 g. carbohydrate = 4 calories
- 1 g. fat = 9 calories

In other words, protein and carbohydrate have the same gram-for-gram calorie count.

It is also thought that protein can burn up fat. This is another erroneous assumption that leaves dieters staring incomprehensibly at their scales. It just is not true that the more protein you eat the thinner you'll get. And believe it or not, one homemade beef taco or a slice of cheese pizza will give you more protein than two eggs or four slices of bacon or even a whole cup of milk. (Of course, if the taco or pizza is made with all sorts of additives, you're better off taking a cut in protein and sticking with the eggs.)

74. Protein Supplements

Two tablespoons of supplement
equal the protein in a three-ounce steak.

For anyone who isn't able to get his or her daily protein requirement from whole food, protein supplements are helpful. The best formulas are derived from soybeans, which contain all the essential amino acids. They come in liquid and powdered form, are available without carbohydrates or fats, and generally supply about 26 g. of protein an ounce (two tablespoons). That would be about the same amount of protein you get from a three-ounce T-bone.

Supplements can easily be added to beverages and foods. Texturized vegetable protein can be added to ground beef to extend and enhance hamburgers, which will be more economical and better for you because of the cut in saturated fat.

75. Amino Acid Supplements

Free-form amino acids are now available in balanced formulas or as individual supplements, because so many have been found to offer specific health-enhancing properties—from improving the immune system to reducing dependence on drugs. (See individual listings, sections 76 through 82.)

It's wise, when taking amino acid supplements, to also take the major vitamins that are involved in their metabolisms— vitamins B_6, B_{12}, and niacin, for instance. And if you're going to take an amino acid formula, make sure it's well balanced. *Read the label!* For protein synthesis to occur, there must be a balance between "essential" and "nonessential" amino acids, and the essentials must be in proper proportion to one another. (Lysine should be in a 2:1 ratio to methionine, 3:1 to tryptophan, and so on. When in doubt, ask your pharmacist or consult a reliable nutritionist. Or send a stamped, self-addressed envelope, with your question, to Amino Acid Research Group, P.O. Box 5277, Berkeley, CA 94705.) What you want is a formula that's modeled after naturally occurring proteins so that you can get the proper therapeutic value.

CAUTION: It's dangerous for any supplement to be used in place of food on a regular basis, taken in megadoses, or substituted for medication without the advice of a physician. Always keep them out of the reach of children.

76. Let's Talk Tryptophan

Tryptophan is an essential amino acid that's used by the brain—along with vitamin B_6, niacin (or niacinamide), and magnesium—to produce serotonin, a neurotransmitter that carries messages between the brain and one of the body's biochemical mechanisms of sleep.

WHAT IT CAN DO FOR YOU:

Help induce natural sleep.
Reduce pain sensitivity.
Act as a nondrug antidepressant.
Aid in reducing anxiety and tension.
Help relieve some symptoms of alcohol-related body chemistry disorders and aid in control of alcoholism.

BEST NATURAL SOURCES:

Cottage cheese, milk, meat, fish, turkey, bananas, dried dates, peanuts, all protein-rich foods.

SUPPLEMENTS:

L-tryptophan comes in tablets of 250-mg. to 667-mg. strengths. When used as a relaxant, it should be taken during the day between meals, with juice or water—no milk or other protein.

As a sleep inducer, L-tryptophan works best when taken in a 500-mg. dose, along with vitamin B_6 100 mg., niacinamide 100 mg., and chelated magnesium 130 mg., one and one-half hours before bedtime. (Again, these should be taken with juice or water—no protein.)

Many doctors, including Dr. David Bressler, formerly of the Pain Control Center at the University of California, suggest taking an additional tryptophan tablet one-half hour before bedtime to help you sleep all through the night.

CAUTION: Single dosages exceeding 2 grams are not recommended, even though successful tests at the Maryland Psychiatric Research Center have shown that there is no danger of tryptophan addiction or overdose. (Because tryptophan is a natural part of our physical makeup, the body doesn't have to change any function to make use of it as it does with drugs.) If you experience any adverse reaction, discontinue use and consult a physician.

PERSONAL ADVICE:

If you are taking L-tryptophan, be sure that you're also taking a complete balanced B-complex formula (50 to 100 mg. of B_1, B_2, and B_6) with your morning and evening meals.

You can prolong the relaxant effects of tryptophan by taking it in a two-to-one ratio with niacinamide (twice as much tryptophan as niacinamide). Niacinamide has an antidepressant effect of its own. (See section 44.)

77. The Phenomenal Phenylalanine

Phenylalanine is an essential amino acid that is a neuro-transmitter, a chemical that transmits its signals between the nerve cells and the brain. In the body it's turned into norepinephrine and dopamine, excitatory transmitters, which promote alertness and vitality. (Do not confuse with DL-phenylalanine; see section 78.)

WHAT IT CAN DO FOR YOU:

Reduce hunger.
Increase sexual interest.
Improve memory and mental alertness.
Alleviate depression.

BEST NATURAL SOURCES:

All protein-rich foods, bread stuffing, soy products, cottage cheese, dry skim milk, almonds, peanuts, lima beans, pumpkin and sesame seeds.

SUPPLEMENTS:

Available in 250- to 500-mg. tablets. For appetite control, tablets should be taken one hour before meals with juice or water (no protein).

For general alertness and vitality, tablets should be taken between meals, but again with water or juice (no protein.)

CAUTION: Phenylalanine is contraindicated during pregnancy and for people with PKU (phenylketonuria) or skin cancer.

PERSONAL ADVICE:

Before resorting to prescription or recreational drugs, I'd advice giving this natural "upper" a chance. (Keep in mind, though, that it cannot be metabolized if you are deficient in vitamin C.)

Phenylalanine is nonaddictive, *but it can raise blood pressure*. If you are hypertensive or have a heart condition, I'd advise checking with your doctor before using phenylalanine. (In most cases, persons with high blood pressure are able to take phenylalanine *after* meals, but clear it with your doctor first.)

78. DL-Phenylalanine (DLPA)

This form of the essential amino acid phenylalanine is a mixture of equal parts of D (synthetic) and L (natural) phenylalanine. By producing and activating morphinelike hormones called *endorphins,* it intensifies and prolongs the body's own natural painkilling response to injury, accident, and disease.

Certain enzyme systems in the body continually destroy endorphins, but DL-phenylalanine effectively inhibits these enzymes, allowing the painkilling endorphins to do their job.

Many people who do not respond to such
conventional painkillers as Empirin
and codeine *do* respond to DLPA.

People who suffer from chronic pain have lower levels of endorphin activity in their blood and cerebrospinal fluid. Since DLPA can restore normal endorphin levels, it can thereby assist the body in reducing pain naturally—without the use of drugs.

Moreover, because DLPA is capable of selective pain blocking, it can effectively alleviate chronic long-term discomfort while leaving the body's natural defense mechanisms for short-term acute pain (burns, cuts, and the like) unhindered.

The effect of DLPA often equals or exceeds that of morphine and other opiate derivatives, but DLPA differs from prescription and over-the-counter medicines in that . . .

- It is nonaddictive.
- Pain relief becomes *more* effective over time (without development of tolerance).
- It has strong antidepressant action.
- It can provide continuous pain relief for up to a month without additional medication.
- It's nontoxic.
- It can be combined with any other medication or therapy to increase benefits without adverse interactions.

WHAT IT CAN DO FOR YOU:

Act as a natural painkiller for conditions such as whiplash, osteoarthritis, rheumatoid arthritis, lower back pain, migraines, leg and muscle cramps, postoperative pain, and neuralgia.

SUPPLEMENTS:

DL-phenylalanine is generally available in 375-mg. tablets. Correct dosages vary according to the individual's own experience of pain.

Six tablets per day (two tablets taken approximately fifteen minutes before each meal) is the best way to begin a DLPA regimen. Pain relief should occur within the first four days, though it may, in some cases, take as long as three to four weeks. (If no substantial relief is noticed in the first three weeks, double the initial dosage for an additional two to three weeks. If treatment is still not effective, discontinue the regimen. It's been found that 5 to 15 percent of users do not respond to DLPA's analgesic properties.)

CAUTION: DLPA is contraindicated during pregnancy and for people with PKU (phenylketonuria). Because it may elevate blood pressure, people with heart conditions or hypertension should check with a doctor before starting any DLPA regimen. Usually, though, it's allowed if taken *after* meals.

PERSONAL ADVICE:

On a DLPA regimen, pain usually diminishes within the first week. Dosages can then be reduced gradually until a minimum requirement is determined. Whatever yours turns out to be, doses should be regularly spaced throughout the day.

Some people require only one week of DLPA supplements a month; others need it on a continuous basis. (I found it interesting to discover that many people who do not respond to such conventional prescription painkillers as Empirin and codeine *do* respond to DLPA.)

79. Looking at Lysine

This essential amino acid is vital in the makeup of critical body proteins. It's needed for growth, tissue repair, and the production of antibodies, hormones, and enzymes.

WHAT IT CAN DO FOR YOU:

Help reduce the incidence of and/or prevent herpes simplex infection.
Promote better concentration.
Properly utilize fatty acids needed for energy production.
Aid in alleviating some fertility problems.

BEST NATURAL SOURCES:

Fish, milk, lima beans, meat, cheese, yeast, eggs, soy products, all protein-rich foods.

SUPPLEMENTS:

L-lysine is generally available in 500-mg. capsules. The usual dosage is 1 to 2 capsules daily between meals.

PERSONAL ADVICE:

If you're often tired, unable to concentrate, prone to bloodshot eyes, nausea, dizziness, hair loss, and anemia, you could have a lysine deficiency.

Older persons, particularly men, require more lysine than younger ones.

Lysine is lacking in certain cereal proteins such as gliadin (from wheat) and zein (from corn). Supplementation of wheat-based foods with lysine improves their protein quality. (See complete and incomplete protein in section 72.)

If you have cold sores or other herpes simplex infection, lysine supplements in doses of 3 to 6 grams daily—plus lysine-rich foods—are strongly recommended. Take between meals, with water (no protein).

80. All About Arginine

This amino acid is necessary for the normal function of the pituitary gland. Along with ornithine, phenylalanine, and other neurochemicals, arginine is required for the synthesis and release of the pituitary gland's growth hormone. (See section 81.) The need for arginine is especially great in males, since seminal fluids contain as much as 80 percent of this protein building block, and a deficiency could lead to infertility.

WHAT IT CAN DO FOR YOU:

Increase sperm count in males.
Aid in immune response and healing of wounds.
Help metabolize stored body fat and tone up muscle tissue.

BEST NATURAL SOURCES:

Nuts, popcorn, carob, gelatin desserts, chocolate, brown rice, oatmeal, raisins, sunflower and sesame seeds, whole-wheat bread, and all protein-rich foods.

SUPPLEMENTS:

L-arginine is available in tablets or powder. It's best taken on an empty stomach (with water) in a 2-gram (2,000-mg.) dose immediately before retiring. Additional benefits—particularly those for muscle toning—can be gained by taking 2 grams (2,000 mg.) on an empty stomach (with water) one hour prior to engaging in vigorous physical exercise.

CAUTION: Do not give to growing children (could cause giantism) or persons with schizophrenic conditions. Arginine supplements—and arginine-rich foods—are contraindicated for anyone who has herpes. Dosages exceeding 20 to 30 grams daily are not recommended (could cause enlarged joints and deformities of bones).

PERSONAL ADVICE:

Arginine is necessary for adults because after the age of thirty there is almost a complete cessation of its secretion from the pituitary gland.

If you notice a thickening or coarsening of your skin, you're taking too much arginine. Several weeks of extremely high doses can cause this side effect, but it is reversible. Just cut back on your intake.

Any physical trauma increases your need for dietary arginine.

L-arginine taken in conjunction with L-ornithine can help stimulate weight loss.

81. Growth Hormone (G.H.) Releasers

Growth hormone (G.H.) releasers are nutrients that stimulate the production of growth hormone in the body. The human growth hormone is stored in the pituitary gland and the body releases it in response to sleep, exercise, and restricted food intake.

WHAT IT CAN DO FOR YOU:

Help burn fat and convert it into energy and muscle.
Improve resistance to disease.
Accelerate wound healing.
Aid in tissue repair.
Strengthen connective tissue for healthier tendons and ligaments.
Enhance protein synthesis for muscle growth.
Reduce urea levels in blood and urine.

Important G.H. releasers are the amino acids ornithine, arginine, tryptophan, glycine, and tyrosine, which work synergistically (more effectively together than separately) with vitamin B_6, niacinamide, zinc, calcium, magnesium, potassium, and vitamin C to trigger the nighttime release of growth hormone. Peak secretion of G.H. is reached about ninety minutes after we fall asleep.

Natural growth hormone levels decrease as we grow older. Somewhere around age fifty, G.H. production stops completely. But by supplementing your diet with amino acids and vitamins that stimulate release of growth hormone, production can be brought back up to the level of a young adult.

CAUTION: Diabetics are not advised to take growth hormones because they may interfere with necessary insulin distribution. Also, no one under the age of twenty-five should take growth hormones, unless they have been specifically prescribed by a physician.

THE DYNAMIC AMINO DUO: ORNITHINE AND ARGININE

Ornithine and arginine, two of the amino acids involved in the release of human growth hormone, are among the most popular amino acid supplements today, essentially because they can help you slim down and shape up while you sleep (which is when G.H. is secreted). While some hormones encourage the body to store fat, growth hormone acts as a mobilizer of fat, helping you not only to look trimmer but to have more energy as well.

Ornithine stimulates insulin secretion and helps insulin work as an anabolic (muscle-building) hormone, which has increased its use among body builders. Taking extra ornithine will help increase the levels of arginine in your body. (Actually, arginine is constructed from ornithine and ornithine is released from arginine in a continuing cyclic process.)

Because ornithine and arginine are so closely related, the characteristics and cautions for one apply to the other. (See section 80, "All About Arginine.") As a supplement, ornithine works best when taken at the same time and in the same manner as arginine (on an empty stomach, with water—no protein).

82. Other Amazing Amino Acids

GLUTAMINE AND GLUTAMIC ACID

Glutamic acid serves primarily as a brain fuel. It has the ability to pick up excess ammonia—which can inhibit high-performance brain function—and convert it into the buffer glutamine. Since glutamine produces marked elevation of glutamic acid, a shortage of the former in the diet can result in a shortage of the latter in the brain.

Aside from improving intelligence (even the IQs of mentally deficient children), glutamine has been shown to help in the control of alcoholism. It has also been found to shorten the healing time for ulcers and alleviate fatigue, depression, and impotence. Most recently it's been used successfully in the treatment of schizophrenia and senility.

L-glutamine (the natural form of glutamine) is available as a supplement in 500-mg. capsules. The recommended dosage is 1 to 4 grams (1,000 to 4,000 mg.) daily, in divided doses. (For fatigue, depression, and impotence, the recommended dosage is 500 to 1,000 mg. daily for the first few weeks, 1,200 to 1,500 mg. for the next few weeks, and finally 2,000 mg. after a month.)

CAUTION: Though glutamine and glutamic acid are not the same as monosodium glutamate (MSG), persons with a sensitivity to the latter could experience an allergic reaction and are advised to consult a physician before using these supplements.

ASPARTIC ACID

Aspartic acid aids in the expulsion of harmful ammonia from the body. (When ammonia enters the circulatory system, it acts as a highly toxic substance.) By disposing of ammonia, aspartic acid helps protect the central nervous system. Recent research indicates that it may be an important factor in increased resistance to fatigue. When salts of aspartic acid were given to athletes, they showed decidedly improved stamina and endurance.

L-aspartic acid (the natural form of aspartic acid) is available as a supplement in 250-mg. and 500-mg. tablets. The usual dosage is 500 mg. 1 to 3 times daily with juice or water (no protein).

CYSTINE AND CYSTEINE

Cystine is the *stable form* of the sulfur-containing amino acid cysteine (an important antiaging nutrient). The body readily converts one into the other as needed, and the two forms can be considered as a single amino acid in metabolism. When cystine is metabolized, it yields sulfuric acid, which reacts with other substances to help detoxify the system.

Sulfur-containing amino acids, particularly cystine and methionine, have been shown to be effective protectors against copper toxicity. (An excessive accumulation of copper in humans is a sign of Wilson's disease.) Cystine/cysteine can also help "tie up" and protect the body from other harmful metals as well as destructive free radicals that are formed by smoking and drinking. A cysteine supplement taken daily with vitamin C (*three times as much vitamin C as cysteine*) is the regimen that's been suggested for smokers and alcohol drinkers. (Supplements need not be taken on an empty stomach.) Recent research also indicates that therapeutic doses of cysteine can offer an important degree of protection against X-ray and nuclear radiation.

CAUTION: Large doses of cysteine/cystine, vitamin C, and vitamin B_1 are not recommended for anyone with diabetes mellitus and should only be taken on the advice of a physician. (The combination of these nutrients could negate insulin effectiveness.)

METHIONINE

Like cysteine, this is another sulfur-containing amino acid. Methionine helps in some cases of schizophrenia by lowering the blood level of histamine, which can cause the brain to relay wrong messages. When combined with choline and folic acid, it has been shown to offer protection against certain tumors.

An insufficiency of methionine can break down the body's ability to process urine and result in edema (swelling due to retention of fluids in tissues) and susceptibility to infection. A methionine deficiency in laboratory animals has been linked to cholesterol deposits, atherosclerosis, and hair loss.

GLYCINE

Sometimes referred to as the simplest of the amino acids, glycine has been shown to yield quite a few remarkable benefits. It has been found helpful in the treatment of low pituitary gland function, and, because it supplies the body with additional creatine (essential for muscle function), it has also been found effective in the treatment of progressive muscular dystrophy.

Many nutritionally oriented doctors now use glycine in the treatment of hypoglycemia. (Glycine stimulates the release of glucagon, which mobilizes glycogen, which is then released into the blood as glucose.)

Additionally, it is effective as a treatment for gastric hyperacidity (and is included in many gastric antacid drugs). It has also been used to treat certain types of acidemia (low pH of the blood), especially one caused by a leucine imbalance which results in an offensive body and breath odor (a condition formerly treated only by a dietary restriction of leucine).

TYROSINE

Though this is a nonessential amino acid, it's a high-ranking neurotransmitter, and important because of its role in stimulating and modifying brain activity. For instance, in order for phenylalanine to be effective as a mood elevator, appetite depressant, and so forth (see section 77), it must first convert into tyrosine. If this conversion does not take place, either because of some enzyme insufficiency or a great need elsewhere in the body for phenylalanine, insufficient quantities of norepinephrine will be produced by the brain and depression will result.

Clinical studies have shown that tyrosine supplementation has helped control medication-resistant depression and anxiety and enables patients taking amphetamines (as mood elevators or diet drugs) to reduce their dosages to minimal levels in a matter of weeks.

Tyrosine has also helped cocaine addicts kick their habit by helping to avert the depression, fatigue, and extreme irritability that accompany withdrawal. A regimen of tyrosine, dissolved in orange juice, taken along with vitamin C, tyrosine hydroxlase (the enzyme that lets the body use tyrosine), vitamin B_1, vitamin B_2, and niacin seems to work.

83. Any Questions About Chapter V?

I'm prone to convulsions, and my doctor put me on Dilantin (phenytoin) a year ago. Recently, a friend told me about taurine, which she said was a nonessential amino acid that was natural and could help me the same way. What I want to know is, if it's nonessential, why would I need it? And why would it work?

Let me begin by clearing up a major point of misunderstanding: Where amino acids are concerned, nonessential does *not* mean unnecessary. All the amino acids are necessary, it's just that the ones that are deemed essential can't be synthesized by the body in sufficient quantities to promote effective protein synthesis. If these essential ones are not supplied in the diet, *all* amino acids are reduced in the same proportion as the one that's low or missing. As for substituting taurine for an anticonvulsant medication, that's a decision only your doctor can make. I can say, though, that taurine has been shown to be quite successful as an anticonvulsant when taken in combination with glutamic and aspartic acids, but I would not recommend undertaking it without consulting a doctor. (For listings of nutritionally oriented doctors in your area, see section 278.)

I've read that exercise stimulates the release of growth hormone. I do at least twenty minutes of dance exercise every day, so does this mean that I probably don't need a G.H. supplement?

On the contrary, you probably do. Only certain exercises, such as weight lifting, where there is what's known as muscular "peak output" (even briefly sustained), promote a significant release of G.H. Other exercises, even prolonged ones, produce negligible amounts (if any) of growth hormone—unless they are performed with peak muscular effort. In fact, because amino acids are lost through the skin when you sweat, exercise *increases* your need for amino acids that will stimulate growth hormone.

I take Dexatrim to control my weight. On the label it says that it contains phenylpropanolamine. Is this the same as L-phenylalanine, and are they equally effective?

Phenylpropanolamine (PPA), which is found in many diet pills, is definitely *not* the same as L-phenylalanine. PPA is an appetite depressant (of dubious effectiveness, according to the American Medical Association) with a high incidence of side effects, including adverse interactions with MAO inhibitors and some oral contraceptives. Unlike the amino acid phenylalanine, which stimulates the brain to produce norepinephrine (which has been shown to reduce hunger) and alleviate those down-in-the-dumps diet blues, PPA depletes the brain of norepinephrine—usually in about two weeks—and leaves dieters fatigued and often depressed.

PPA is a poor substitute for a good diet (see section 117) while L-phenylalanine, found naturally in such protein-rich foods as cottage cheese, soy products, almonds, dry skim milk, and many more, can aid in appetite control (while nourishing the brain) if taken one hour before meals with juice or water.

Is there such a thing as an antiaging amino acid?

As a matter of fact, L-glutathione (GSH) has been called a triple threat antiaging amino acid. It's actually a tripeptide, synthesized from three amino acids—L-cysteine, L-glutamic acid, and glycine—and it has been shown to act as an antioxidant and deactivate free radicals which speed up the aging process. It is also an antitumor agent and respiratory accelerator in the brain; has been used in the treatment of allergies, cataracts, diabetes, hypoglycemia, and arthritis; helps to prevent the harmful side effects of high-dose radiation in chemotherapy and X rays; and protects against the harmful effects of cigarette smoke and alcohol.

What is this new amino acid L-carnitine that I have been hearing about?

We're all very excited about it, since recent research has indicated that not only does it play an important role in converting stored body fat into energy, but it can also help control hypoglycemia, reduce angina attacks, and benefit patients with diabetes, liver disease, or kidney disease.

The heart is dependent upon L-carnitine, and a deficiency of this amino acid can cause impairment of heart tissue. The major natural sources are meats and dairy products.

With diseases such as cancer, AIDS, and what-have-you on the rampage these days, is there anything that can be done to improve an individual's immune system?

Fortunately, yes! The answer seems to be growth hormone releasers (see section 81).

What happens is that as we get older, our immune system—that ever-ready army of white blood cells (called T cells because they're under the command of the thymus gland) which are told where and when to attack and what antibodies their cofighters (called B cells because they're made in the bone marrow) should produce—begins to break down due to the decreasing power and size of the thymus gland. This not only causes an ineffectual defense system, but can create a dangerous confusion where the T cells mistake friends for enemies and attack you, resulting in autoimmune disorders. (It's been suggested that diseases such as multiple sclerosis, myasthenia gravis, and arthritis may be caused by this.)

What's been discovered recently, though, is that this breakdown is most likely the result of a reduced rate of growth hormone, which is produced by the pituitary gland and is necessary to the function of the thymus gland and therefore the immune system. But supplements of amino acids (arginine, ornithine, and cysteine), as well as vitamins E, A, C, zinc, selenium, and enzymes such as papain, have been found to work wonders in reversing this degenerative syndrome.

VI

Fat and Fat Manipulators

84. Lipotropics—What Are They?

Methionine, choline, inositol, and betaine are all lipotropics, which means their prime function is to prevent abnormal or excessive accumulation of fat in the liver.

Lipotropics also increase the liver's production of lecithin, which keeps cholesterol more soluble; detoxify the liver; and increase resistance to disease by helping the thymus gland carry out its functions.

85. Who Needs Them and Why

We all need lipotropics, some of us more than others. Anyone on a high-protein diet falls into the latter category. Methionine and choline are *necessary* to detoxify the amines that are by-products of protein metabolism.

Because nearly all of us consume too much fat (the average consumption in the United States is now 40 to 45 percent of total calories), and a good part of that is saturated fat, lipotropics are indispensable. By helping the liver produce lecithin, they're helping to keep cholesterol from forming dangerous deposits in blood vessels, lessening chances of heart attacks, arteriosclerosis, and gallstone formation.

> Lipotropics keep cholesterol
> moving safely.

We also need lipotropics to stay healthy, since they aid the thymus in stimulating the production of antibodies, promoting the growth and action of phagocytes (which surround and gobble up invading viruses and microbes), and destroying foreign or abnormal tissue.

86. The Cholesterol Story

Like everything else, there's a good and bad side to fats. The general misconception that all of them are bad for you, prevalent as it may be, is simply not true. And cholesterol is the most maligned fat of all.

Practically everyone knows that cholesterol can be responsible for arteriosclerosis, heart attacks, a variety of illnesses, but very few are aware of the ways in which it is *essential* to health.

At least two-thirds of your body cholesterol is produced by the liver or in the intestine. It is found there as well as in the brain, the adrenals, and nerve fiber sheaths. And when it's good, it's very, very good:

• Cholesterol in the skin is converted to essential vitamin D when touched by the sun's ultraviolet rays.

• Cholesterol aids in the metabolism of carbohydrates. (The more carbohydrates ingested, the more cholesterol produced.)

• Cholesterol is a prime supplier of life-essential adrenal steroid hormones, such as cortisone, and of sex hormones.

New research shows that cholesterol behaves differently depending on the protein to which it is bound. Lipoproteins are the factors in our blood that transport cholesterol. Low-density lipoproteins (LDL) carry about 65 percent of blood cholesterol, very-low-density lipoproteins (VLDL) about 15 percent, and they do seem to bear a correlation to heart disease. But high-density lipoproteins (HDL), which carry about 20 percent, appear to have the opposite effect. HDL are composed principally of lecithin, whose detergent action breaks up cholesterol and can transport it easily through the blood without clogging arteries. Essentially, the higher your HDL, the lower your chances of developing symptoms of heart disease.

It's interesting to note that females, who live eight years longer than males on the average, have higher HDL levels, and, surprisingly, so do moderate alcohol drinkers.

> Eggs might not be as bad
> as you thought.

It is also worth mentioning that though the egg consumption in the United States is one-half of what it was in 1945, there has *not* been a comparable decline in heart disease. And though the American Heart Association deems eggs hazardous, a diet without them can be equally hazardous. Not only do eggs have the most perfect protein components of any food, but they contain lecithin, which aids in fat assimilation. Most important, they *raise* HDL levels!

87. How to Raise and Lower Cholesterol Levels

RAISE CHOLESTEROL	LOWER CHOLESTEROL
Cigarettes	Eggplant
Food additives such as BHT	Onions (raw or cooked—but not fried)
Pollutants such as PCBs	Garlic
Coffee	Yogurt (even made from whole milk)
Stress	Pectin (unpeeled apple, scraped
The pill	apple, white membrane of citrus
Refined sugar	fruits)
Saturated fats	Soybeans
	Carrots (raw)
	Fiber
	Pinto, navy, and kidney beans
	Polyunsaturated oils
	Chromium supplements
	Vitamins C, E, and niacin
	Lecithin lipotropics

For cholesterol watchers, a meal of light meat turkey is a good choice, especially since no more than 300 mg. of cholesterol a day are recommended for the average person. Three ounces of light meat turkey has only about 67 mg. cholesterol (though the same amount of dark meat has 75 mg.). Be careful of turkey liver, though; one cup of it, chopped, has about 839 mg. And remember, vegetables are cholesterol-free without butter.

88. Any Questions About Chapter VI?

Are lipotropics available as supplements, and if so, what's the recommended dosage and are there any special instructions for taking them?

Lipotropics are available as supplements in tablet form. (Usually 3 tablets equal 1,000 mg.—or 1 gram—of each lipotropic agent.) The dosage most often recommended is 1 to 2 tablets taken 3 times daily, *with* food.

Do you consider lipotropic supplements more important for some people than others?

Definitely, especially since studies have shown that Americans eat 100 pounds of fat per person a year, and lipotropics are the substances that can liquefy or homogenize fats. I feel that supplementation is particularly important for anyone on a high-protein diet, because lipotropics detoxify amines, which are by-products of protein metabolism. Also, anyone worried about gallstone formation would be wise to consider these supplements.

Is it really so important to use polyunsaturated oils?

Only if you care about keeping your cholesterol levels down and perhaps staving off heart attacks and high blood pressure, among other things.

Polyunsaturated fats are vegetable oils (sunflower, corn, safflower, and soy, for example). These have shown definite evidence of lowering blood serum cholesterol. Saturated fat, as well as hydrogenated and even partially hydrogenated oils, can cause just the opposite. It's a good idea to read labels carefully. For instance, when buying margarine, make sure the first ingredient reads polyunsaturated vegetable oil. The second ingredient will undoubtedly be a partially hydrogenated oil, but at least it's in second place. The more you can decrease your consumption of saturated fats, minimize your intake of hydrogenated fats, and increase the polyunsaturates in your diet, the better off you'll be.

Avoid peanut, coconut, and palm oils; take vitamin E (400 to 800 IU daily) to help prevent lipid peroxidation (fats "rusting" in the body); increase the amount of fish—such as mackerel and cod—you eat; and don't forget to drink plenty of water daily.

VII
Carbohydrates and Enzymes

89. Why Carbohydrates Are Necessary

Carbohydrates, the scourge of misinformed dieters, are the main suppliers of our body's energy. During digestion, starches and sugars—the principal kinds of carbohydrates—are broken down into glucose, better known as blood sugar. This blood sugar provides the essential energy for our brain and central nervous system.

You need carbohydrates in your daily diet so that vital tissue-building protein is not wasted for energy when it might be needed for repair.

> They have the same calories
> as protein.

If you eat too many carbohydrates, more than can be converted into glucose or glycogen (which is stored in the liver and muscles), the result, as we know all too well, is fat. When the body needs more fuel, the fat is converted back to glucose and you lose weight.

Don't be too down on carbohydrates. They're as important for good health as other nutrients—and gram for gram they have the same 4 calories as protein. Though no official requirement exists, a minimum of 50 g. daily is recommended to avoid ketosis, an acid condition of the blood that can happen when your own fat is used primarily for energy.

90. The Truth About Enzymes

Enzymes are necessary for the digestion of food; they release valuable vitamins, minerals, and amino acids, which keep us alive and healthy.

Enzymes are catalysts, meaning they have the power to cause an internal action without themselves being changed or destroyed in the process.

Enzymes are destroyed under certain heat conditions.

Enzymes are best obtained from uncooked or unprocessed fruits, vegetables, eggs, meats, and fish.

Each enzyme acts upon a specific food; one cannot substitute for the other. A deficiency, shortage, or even the absence of one single enzyme can mean the difference between sickness and health.

Enzymes that end in *-ase* are named by the food substance they act upon. For example, with phosphorus the enzyme is called phosphatase; with sugar (sucrose) it is known as sucrase.

Pepsin is a vital digestive enzyme that breaks up the proteins of ingested food, splitting them into usable amino acids. Without pepsin, protein could not be used to build healthy skin, strong skeletal structure, rich blood supply, and strong muscles.

Renin is a digestive enzyme that causes coagulation of milk, changing its protein, casein, into a usable form in the body. Renin releases the valuable minerals from milk—calcium, phosphorus, potassium, and iron—that are used by the body to stabilize the water balance, strengthen the nervous system, and produce strong teeth and bones.

Lipase splits fat, which is then utilized to nourish the skin cells, protect the body against bruises and blows, and ward off the entrance of infectious virus cells and allergic conditions.

Hydrochloric acid in the stomach works on tough foods such as fibrous meats, vegetables, and poultry. It digests protein, calcium, and iron. Without HCl, problems such as pernicious anemia, gastric carcinoma, congenital achlorhydria, and allergies can develop. Because stress, tension, anger, and anxiety before eating, as well as deficiencies of some vitamins (B complex primarily) and minerals, can all cause a lack of HCl, more of us are short of hydrochloric acid than realize it. If you think that you have an overacid problem or heartburn, for which you are dosing yourself with an antacid such as Maalox, Di-Gel, Tums, Rolaids, or Alka-Seltzer, you are probably unaware that *the symptoms of having too little acid are exactly the same as having too much*, in which case the taking of antacids could be the worst possible thing for you to do.

Dr. Alan Nittler, author of *A New Breed of Doctor,* has stated emphatically that everyone over the age of forty should be using an HC1 supplement. Betaine HC1 and glutamic acid HCl are the best forms of commercially available hydrochloric acid.

CAUTION: If you have an ulcer condition, consult your doctor before using these supplements.

91. The Twelve Tissue Salts and Their Functions

Tissue salts are inorganic mineral components of your body's tissues. They are also known as Schuessler biochemical cell salts, after Dr. W. H. Schuessler, who isolated them in the late nineteenth century. Dr. Schuessler found that if the body was deficient in any of these salts, illness occurred, and that if the deficiency was corrected, the body could heal itself. In other words, tissue salts are *not a cure,* merely a remedy.

The twelve tissue salts are:

Fluoride of lime (calc. flour.) Part of all the connective tissues in your body. An imbalance can be the cause of varicose veins, late dentition, muscle tendon strain, carbuncles, and cracked skin.

Phosphate of lime (calc. phos.) Found in all your body's cells and fluids, an important element in gastric juices as well as bones and teeth. An imbalance or deficiency can be the cause of cold hands and feet, numbness, hydrocele, sore breasts, and night sweats.

Sulfate of lime (calc. sulf.) A constituent of all connective tissue in minute particles, as well as in the cells of the liver. An imbalance or deficiency can be the cause of skin eruptions, deep abscesses, or chronic oozing ulcers.

Phosphate of iron (ferr. phos.) Part of your blood and other body cells, with the exception of nerves. An imbalance or deficiency can be the cause of continuous diarrhea or, paradoxically, constipation. It has also been used as a remedy for nosebleeds and excessive menses.

Chloride of potash (kali. mur.) Found in lining and under the surface body cells. An imbalance or deficiency can be the cause of granulation of the eyelids, blistering eczema, and warts.

Sulfate of potash (kali. sulf.). The cells that form your skin and internal organ linings interact with this salt. An imbalance or deficiency can be the cause of skin eruptions, a yellow coating on the back of the tongue, feelings of heaviness, and pains in the limbs.

Potassium phosphate (kali. phos.) Found in all your body tissues, particularly nerve, brain, and blood cells. An imbalance or deficiency can be the cause of improper fat digestion, poor memory, anxiety, insomnia, and a faint, rapid pulse.

Phosphate of magnesia (mag. phos.) Another mineral element of bones, teeth, brain, nerves, blood, and muscle cells. An imbalance or deficiency can be the cause of cramps, neuralgia, shooting pains, and colic.

Chloride of soda (nat. mur.) Regulates the amount of moisture in the body and carries moisture to cells. An imbalance or deficiency can be the cause of salt cravings, hay fever, watery discharges from the eyes and nose.

Phosphate of soda (nat. phos.) Emulsifies fatty acids and keeps uric acid soluble in the blood. An imbalance or deficiency can be the cause of jaundice, sour breath, an acid or coppery taste in the mouth.

Sulfate of soda (nat. sulf). A slight irritant to tissues and functions as a stimulant for natural secretions. An imbalance or deficiency can be the cause of low fevers, edema, depression, and gallbladder disorders.

Silicic acid (silicea) Part of all connective tissue cells, as well as those of the hair, nails, and skin. A deficiency or imbalance can be the cause of poor memory, carbuncles, falling hair, and ribbed, ingrowing nails. Eating whole-grain products should supply the normal need for this tissue salt.

92. Any Questions About Chapter VII?

My father-in-law suffers terribly from heartburn and takes Maalox so often that it's virtually his dessert after meals. Isn't there some natural alternative?

There sure is, and it tastes a lot better than any chalky liquid. Chewable papaya enzyme tablets, made from nature's "magic melon" fruit, can actually digest 2,230 times their weight of starch. They do this because they contain papain and prolase, enzymes that assist in protein digestion and combine with mylase, a potent starch digestive enzyme. (Papain, by the way, is the chief ingredient in meat tenderizers, which work on foods before they even reach your stomach.) The U.S. Department of Agriculture has attested to the fact that papaya contains valuable digestive properties, so your father-in-law would be well advised (and probably a lot happier) to take one or two of these pleasant-tasting natural tablets after his meals.

VIII
Other Wonder Workers

93. Acidophilus

Lactobacillus acidophilus, or acidophilus, as it is commonly known, is a source of friendly intestinal bacteria and more effective than yogurt. It is available as acidophilus culture, incubated in soy, milk, or yeast bases.

> Regular use of acidophilus keeps
> the intestines clean.

Many doctors prescribe acidophilus in conjunction with oral antibiotic treatment because antibiotics destroy beneficial intestinal flora, often causing diarrhea as well as an overgrowth of the fungus *Candida albicans*. This fungus can grow in the intestines, vagina, lungs, mouth (thrush), on the fingers, or under the nails. It will usually disappear after a few days' use of generous amounts of acidophilus culture.

Regular use of acidophilus culture keeps the intestines clean. It can eliminate bad breath caused by intestinal putrefaction (the sort resistant to mouthwash or breath spray), constipation, foul-smelling flatulence, and aid in the treatment of acne and other skin problems.

Keep in mind that lactose, complex carbohydrates, pectin, and vitamin C plus roughage encourage additional growth of intestinal flora. This is important since friendly bacteria can die within five days unless they are continuously supplied with some form of lactic acid or lactose—like acidophilus.

94. Ginseng

It is generally well accepted that ginseng is a stimulant of both mental and physical energy. The Chinese have been using it for nearly five thousand years and still revere it as a preventive and cure-all. It is a mild laxative and helps the body pass poisons through more rapidly. Its reputed benefits include cures for impotence, high and low blood pressure, anemia, arthritis, indigestion, insomnia, fatigue, hypoglycemia, poor circulation, and more.

Miracles aside, ginseng does help you assimilate vitamins and minerals by acting as an endocrine-gland stimulant. It is best to take it on an empty stomach, preferably before breakfast, if you want it to be most effective.

Vitamin C has been said to neutralize part of ginseng's value, but there is no real evidence to support this. (If you take a vitamin-C supplement, the time-release form makes counteraction less likely.)

Ginseng is available in capsule form, under names such as Siberian ginseng and Korean ginseng, in 500- to 650-mg. (10-grain) doses. It can also be purchased as tea, liquid concentrate, or as ginseng root in a bottle.

95. Alfalfa, Garlic, Chlorophyll, and Yucca

A natural diuretic

Alfalfa has been dubbed "the great healer" by noted biologist and author Frank Bouer, who discovered that the green leaves of this remarkable legume contain *eight* essential enzymes. Also, for every 100 g., it contains 8,000 IU of vitamin A and 20,000 to 40,000 units of vitamin K, which protects against hemorrhaging and helps in blood clotting. It is additionally a fine source of vitamins B_6 and E, and it contains enough vitamin D, lime, and phosphorus to secure strong bones and teeth in growing children.

Many doctors have used alfalfa in treating stomach ailments, gas pains, ulcerous conditions, and poor appetite, because it contains vitamin U, which is also found in raw cabbage and cabbage juice. The latter has frequently been used as an aid in treating peptic ulcers. Alfalfa is also a good laxative and a natural diuretic.

"Russian penicillin"

Garlic contains potassium, phosphorus, a significant amount of B and C vitamins, calcium, and protein. In Europe it is respected as a valuable medicine. The Soviets call it "Russian penicillin." In America it is virtually ignored.

Despite its small acceptance here, it does appear to have some amazing properties. Many medical authorities feel that it can reduce high blood pressure by either neutralizing the poisonous substances in the intestines or acting as a vasodilator. F. G. Piotrousky, of the University of Vienna, found that 40 percent of his hypertensive patients had substantially lower blood pressure after they were given garlic.

Garlic has also been found to be effective in cleaning the blood of excess glucose. (Blood sugar ranks with cholesterol as a causative factor in arteriosclerosis and heart attacks.) This is not to suggest, though, that it be used to replace medically prescribed methods. In addition, it has also been reported to alleviate grippe, sore throat, and bronchial congestion.

The best way to take garlic as a supplement is in the form of perles. These caps contain the valuable garlic oils and leave no after-odor on the breath, because they do not dissolve in the stomach but in the lower digestive tract. Garlic tablets with parsley (which contains natural chlorophyll) are also available.

Chlorophyll, according to G. W. Rapp in the *American Journal of Pharmacy,* possesses positive antibacterial action. It also appears to act as a wound-healing agent, and, while stimulating the growth of new tissue, it reduces the hazard of bacterial contamination.

Nature's deodorant, chlorophyll is used in commercial air fresheners, as a topical body deodorant, and as an oral breath refresher. It is available in tablets and in liquid preparations.

Yucca extract comes from the genus of trees and shrubs belonging to the Liliaceae family (the Joshua tree is a yucca). The Indians used the yucca for many purposes and revered it as a plant that guaranteed their health and survival. Dr. John W. Yale, a botanical biochemist, extracted the steroid saponin from the plant and used the extract in a tablet for the treatment of arthritis. The treatment proved safe and effective (the average dose was four tablets daily), and there was no gastrointestinal irritation. Yucca-extract tablets are nontoxic and available in most health-food and vitamin stores.

96. Fiber and Bran

When research appeared in the *Journal of the American Medical Association* indicating that we would all be a great deal healthier and live longer if we ate coarser diets that sent more indigestible dietary fiber through our digestive tracts, a lot of people, wisely, jumped on the fiber bandwagon, though most weren't aware (and still aren't) that all fiber is not the same and that different types perform different functions.

TYPES OF FIBER YOU SHOULD KNOW ABOUT

Cellulose This is found in whole-wheat flour, bran, cabbage, young peas, green beans, wax beans, broccoli, brussels sprouts, cucumber skins, peppers, apples, and carrots.

Hemicelluloses These are found in bran, cereals, whole grains, brussels sprouts, mustard greens, and beet root.

Cellulose and hemicelluloses absorb water and can smooth functioning of the large bowel. Essentially, they "bulk" waste and move it through the colon more rapidly. This not only can prevent constipation, but may also protect against diverticulosis, spastic colon, hemorrhoids, cancer of the colon, and varicose veins.

Gums These are usually found in oatmeal and other rolled-oat products as well as in dried beans.

Pectin This is found in apples, citrus fruits, carrots,

cauliflower, cabbage, dried peas, green beans, potatoes, squash, and strawberries.

Gums and pectin primarily influence absorption in the stomach and small bowel. By binding with bile acids, they decrease fat absorption and lower cholesterol levels. They delay stomach-emptying by coating the lining of the gut, and by so doing they slow sugar absorption after a meal, which is helpful to diabetics since it reduces the amount of insulin needed at any one time.

Lignin This type of fiber is found in many breakfast cereals, bran, older vegetables (when vegetables age, their lignin content rises and they become less digestible), eggplant, green beans, strawberries, pears, and radishes.

Lignin reduces the digestibility of other fibers. It also binds with bile acids to lower cholesterol and helps speed food through the gut.

CAUTION: While it's true that most of us still don't have enough fiber in our diet, too much can cause gas, bloating, nausea, vomiting, and diarrhea and may possibly interfere with your body's ability to absorb certain minerals, such as zinc, calcium, iron, magnesium, and vitamin B_{12}. This is easily prevented by varying your diet along with your high-fiber foods.

97. Kelp

This amazing seaweed contains more vitamins and minerals than any other food. To be more specific, kelp has vitamin B_2, niacin, choline, carotene, and alginic acid, as well as twenty-three minerals, which range as follows:

Iodine	0.15–0.20%	Magnesium	0.76%
Calcium	1.20%	Sulfur	0.93%
Phosphorus	0.30%	Chlorine	12.21%
Iron	0.10%	Copper	0.0008%
Sodium	3.14%	Zinc	0.0003%
Potassium	0.63%	Manganese	0.0008%

Plus traces of barium, boron, chromium, lithium, nickel, silver, titanium, vanadium, aluminum, strontium, and silicon.

Because of its natural iodine content, kelp has a normalizing effect on the thyroid gland. In other words, thin people with thyroid trouble can gain weight by using kelp, and obese people can lose weight with it.

Homeopathic physicians use kelp for obesity, poor digestion, flatulence, and obstinate constipation; and, for the past several years, one of the most widespread fads has been the kelp, lecithin, vinegar, and B$_6$ diet (see section 249).

98. Yeast

One of the richest sources of
organic iron

It's known as nature's wonder food, and it does a lot to deserve its reputation. Yeast is an excellent source of protein and a superior source of the natural B-complex vitamins. It is one of the richest sources of organic iron and a gold mine of minerals, trace minerals, and amino acids. It has been known to help lower cholesterol (when combined with lecithin), help reverse gout, and ease the aches and pains of neuritis.

There are various sources of yeast:

Brewer's yeast (from hops, a by-product of beer), sometimes called nutritional yeast.

Torula yeast, grown on wood pulp used in the manufacture of paper or produced from blackstrap molasses.

Whey, a by-product of milk and cheese (best-tasting and most potent).

Liquid yeast (from Switzerland and Germany), fed on herbs, honey malt, and oranges or grapefruit.

Avoid live baker's yeast! Live yeast cells deplete the B vitamins in the intestines and rob your body of all vitamins. In nutritional yeast, these live cells are heat-killed, thus preventing that depletion.

Yeast has all the major B vitamins except B_{12}, which can be especially bred into it. It contains sixteen amino acids, fourteen or more minerals, and seventeen vitamins (except for A, E, and C). It can be considered a whole food.

Because yeast, like other protein foods, is high in phosphorus, it is advisable when taking it to add extra calcium to the diet. Phosphorus, though a coworker of calcium, can take calcium out of the body, leaving a deficiency. The remedy is simple: increase your calcium (calcium lactate assimilates well in the body). *B-complex vitamins should be taken together with yeast to be more effective. Together they work like a powerhouse.*

Yeast can be stirred into liquid, juice, or water and taken between meals. Many people who feel fatigued take a tablespoon or more in liquid and feel a return of energy within minutes, and the good effects last for several hours. Yeast can also be used as a reducing food. Stir into liquid and drink just before a meal. It takes the edge off a large appetite and saves you a lot in calories.

99. Any Questions About Chapter VIII?

What's the scoop on spirulina? Is it some sort of wonder drug?

It's not a drug at all. Spirulina is a natural, easily assimilated complete protein. (It's known as spirulina plankton or blue-green algae.) It's nature's highest source of chlorophyll pigment, rich in such chelated minerals as iron, calcium, zinc, potassium, and magnesium, a fine source of vitamin A and B-complex vitamins, and it contains phenylalanine, which acts on the brain's appetite center to decrease hunger pangs—while keeping your blood sugar at the proper level.

If you'd like to slim down, this is a wonderful aid for weight reduction. Take three 500-mg. tablets one-half hour before meals. Once the dosage begins to work, decrease to two or one tablet before meals.

IX

Herbs and Folk Remedies

100. What You Should Know About Natural Remedies

Just because herbs are natural doesn't mean that they can be used indiscriminately. Before trying any herbal remedy, be sure you know what it does, how to prepare and use it—and what cautions or side effects you should be aware of.

Never try any natural or herbal remedy
without knowing what it does, how it should
be prepared and taken, what cautions should
be observed, and what its possible side
effects could be!

As a rule, few medical problems occur from ingesting herbal remedies, but the potential for an allergic or toxic response is always there.

IMPORTANT: If you are now taking any drugs, or have any medical problems, it's wise to consult a nutritionally oriented physician who is aware of herb-drug interactions and any potentially dangerous side effects.

101. Aconite

Small amounts of a fluid extract of the root of this plant mixed in a cup of warm water have been reported to successfully reduce pain, fever, inflammation of the stomach, and heart palpitations.

CAUTION: This is one of the few herbs where misuse can cause a particularly dangerous side effect: heart failure.

102. Aloe Vera

The aloe vera plant contains a wound-healing substance called aloe vera gel, a mixture of antibiotic, astringent, and coagulating agents.

Taken internally, it works as a mild laxative. One tablespoon taken at regular intervals (preferably on an empty stomach) totaling a pint a day, can help in the treatment of stomach ulcers. It is not recommended for pregnant women without the advice of their doctor.

External uses of aloe vera gel are many:

• It acts as an immediate and effective wound healer, aiding in the treatment of burns, insect stings, and poison ivy. Split a leaf and apply pulp directly to the injured area, or soak cloth with aloe vera gel and bind on.

• Aloe vera gel ointments, creams, and lotions can prevent blistering and peeling from sunburn.

• It can help soften corns and calluses on the feet.

• Applied to the face and throat, it can soften skin and hold aging lines in check.

• It can alleviate the pain and itching of hemorrhoids and bleeding piles.

• It can be used as an effective hair conditioner.

CAUTION: Though rare, allergic reactions to aloe vera can occur in sensitive individuals. If you experience any adverse effects, discontinue use and consult a physician.

103. Anise (seed)

This is a natural diuretic and gastric stimulant and is often used to relieve flatulence. It's also been used in home remedies as a treatment for dry cough.

104. Blessed Thistle

Often used as an appetite stimulant and in the treatment of digestive problems, it can reduce fevers and break up congestion.

CAUTION: In high doses, this can cause burns of the mouth and esophagus, as well as diarrhea.

105. Chamomile

This plant has antispasmodic and gastric-stimulant properties and is usually taken internally for migraines, gastric cramps, and anxiety. Externally it's used as a treatment for wounds, skin ulcers, and conjunctivitis.

106. Comfrey

When used in teas, comfrey has been found to alleviate stomach ailments, coughs, diarrhea, arthritis pain, liver problems, and gallbladder conditions.

CAUTION: A possible side effect of using this herb is that it can reduce your absorption of iron and vitamin B_{12}.

107. Juniper (berries)

These are often used as a stomach tonic, can act as appetite and digestion enhancers, and may be helpful as a diuretic and a disinfectant of the urinary tract.

108. Licorice

An effective restorer of membrane and tissue function, it is also a hormone balancer, an intestinal secretion stimulant, a respiratory stimulant, and a laxative.

CAUTION: High blood pressure and cardiac arrhythmias are possible side effects of licorice. (American-manufactured licorice, the sort used in candy, is a synthetic flavoring and does not have these potential side effects—of course, it doesn't offer any of the benefits, either.)

109. Evening Primrose Oil

As a dietary supplement, evening primrose oil can help lower blood cholesterol and blood pressure, help in weight reduction, relieve premenstrual pain, improve eczema, aid in the treatment of moderate cases of rheumatoid arthritis, slow progression of multiple sclerosis, help hyperactive children, improve acne (when taken with zinc), and help build stronger fingernails.

The active ingredient in evening primrose oil is gamma linoleic acid (GLA), which is needed for the body to produce hormonelike compounds called prostaglandins (PGs), vital for good health. In other words, a deficiency of the former can result in impaired production of the latter and adversely affect your physical well-being.

110. Parsley (seeds and leaves)

A diuretic and gastric stimulant, parsley is used medicinally to treat coughs, asthma, amorrhea, dysmenorrhea, and conjunctivitis.

111. Pennyroyal

This herb, often referred to as "lung mint," is used as an inhalant in treating colds; it's also used as a tea for curing headaches, menstrual cramps, and pain.

CAUTION: Pennyroyal can induce abortion and should therefore *never* be used during pregnancy.

112. Peppermint (leaves)

An antispasmodic, tonic, and stimulant, peppermint has been used to treat nervousness, insomnia, cramps, dizziness, and coughs. (For headaches, you might want to try a strong cup of peppermint tea, then lie down for fifteen to twenty minutes. It usually works as effectively as aspirin—and there are *no* side effects.)

113. Rosemary (leaves)

Used externally in an ointment, these can soothe rheumatism aches, sprains, wounds, bruises, and eczema. Taken internally, in the proper preparation, rosemary can relieve flatulence, colic, and stimulate bile release from the gallbladder.

CAUTION: Rosemary can be toxic in large quantities.

114. Thyme

A natural antiseptic and deodorant, thyme—applied externally in compresses—can be an effective liniment for wounds; internally it can act as an antidiarrhetic, relieve gastritis cramps, and soothe bronchitis and laryngitis.

115. Dangerous Herbs

The following herbs can be hazardous to your health and should not be brewed in teas or used in any other fashion because of their potential toxicity.

NOTE: Since many herbs have several common names, the botanical name of the plant is given in italics.

AESCULUS, BUCKEYES, HORSE CHESTNUT (*AESCULUS HIPPOCASANUM*)
   A poisonous plant that contains a toxic coumarin substance.
ARNICA, WOLF'S BANE, LEOPARD'S BANE, MOUNTAIN TOBACCO (*ARNICA MONTANA*)
   Arnica is an irritant and can produce violent toxic gastroenteritis, intense muscular weakness, nervous disorders, and death.
BELLADONNA, DEADLY NIGHTSHADE (*ATROPA BELLADONNA*)
   Poisonous. Contains toxic alkaloids.

BITTERSWEET, DULCAMARA, WOODY OR CLIMBING NIGHTSHADE (*SOLANUM DULCAMARA*)
Poisonous.

BLOODROOT, SANGUINARIA, RED PUCCOON (*SANGUINARIA CANDENSIS*)
Contains the poisonous alkaloid sanguinarine, among others.

BROOM-TOPS, SCOPARIUS, SPARTIUM, IRISH BROOM, SCOTCH BROOM, BROOM (*CYTISUS SCOPARIUS*)
Contains toxic sparteine and other harmful alkaloids.

CALAMUS, SEDGE, SWEET FLAG, SWEET ROOT, SWEET CANE, SWEET CINNAMON (not to be confused with the bark used as a popular spice) (*ACORUS CALAMUS*)
Oil of calamus is a carcinogen (a cancer-causing agent).

HELIOTROPE (*HELIOTROPIUM EUROPAEUM*)
This plant is poisonous and also contains alkaloids that cause liver damage. (It should not be confused with garden heliotrope, whose botanical name is *Valeriana officinalis* and which is safe.)

HEMLOCK, CONIUM, SPOTTED HEMLOCK, SPOTTED PARSLEY, ST. BENNET'S HERB, SPOTTED COWBANE, FOOL'S PARSLEY (*CONIUM MACULATUM*)
Contains poisonous aklaloids. It's often mistaken for water hemlock (*Cicuta virosa* or *maculata*) and hemlock spruce (*Tsuga canadensis*).

HENBANE, HYOSCYAMUS, HOG'S BEAN, POISON TOBACCO, DEVIL'S EYE (*HYOSCYAMUS NIGER*)
Poisonous. Contains dangerously toxic alkaloids.

JALAP ROOT, JALAP BINDWEED, JALAP, TURE

JALAP, VERA CRUZ JALAP, HIGH JOHN ROOT, JOHN CONQUEROR, ST. JOHN THE CONQUEROR ROOT (*EXOGONIUM PURGA, IPOMEA JALAPA, AND IPOMEA PURGA*)

This is a twining Mexican vine known by many different names, but it can be extremely dangerous. The drug is a potent cathartic, and its extreme purgative action can result in life-threatening excessive bowel movements.

JIMSON WEED, DATURA, STRAMONIUM, APPLE OF PERU, JAMESTOWN WEED, THORNAPPLE, TOLGUACHA (*DATURA STRAMONIUM*)

This is a poisonous plant that contains stropine, hyoscyamine, and scopolamine, drugs that are illegal (for good reason) for nonprescription use.

LILY OF THE VALLEY, CONVALLARIA, MAY LILY (*CONVALLARIA MAGALIS*)

A poisonous plant that contains cardiac toxins.

LOBELIA, INDIAN TOBACCO, WILD TOBACCO, ASTHMA WEED, EMETIC WEED (*LOBELIA INFLATA*)

A poisonous plant that is often unwisely used as an emetic. Overdoses of extracts from the plant's leaves or fruit produce severe vomiting, sweating, paralysis, rapid but feeble pulse, and—more often than not—collapse, coma, and death.

MANDRAKE, MANDRAGORA, EUROPEAN MANDRAKE (*MANDRAGORA OFFICINARUM*)

A poisonous narcotic similar to belladonna.

MAY APPLE, MANDRAKE, PODOPHYLLUM, AMERICAN MANDRAKE, DEVIL'S APPLE, UMBRELLA PLANT, VEGETABLE CALOMEL, WILD LEMON, VEGETABLE MERCUTY (*PODOPHYLLUM PELTATUM*)

A poisonous plant with complex toxic constituents.

MISTLETOE, VISCUM, AMERICAN MISTLETOE (*PHORADENDRON FLAVESCENS* AND *VISCUM FLAVESCENS*)

Contains toxic amines. Consider it poisonous.

MISTLETOE, VISCUM, JUNIPER MISTLETOE (*PHORADENDRON JUNIPERINUM*)

This particular mistletoe may or may not be poisonous, but too little is known about it for any wise person to use it for anything but holding up and kissing beneath at Christmastime.

MISTLETOE, VISCUM, EUROPEAN MISTLETOE (*VISCUM ALBUM*)

This branch of mistletoe definitely contains toxic amines and is considered poisonous.

MORNING GLORY (*IPOMEA PURPUREA*)

The seeds of this particular morning glory do contain amides of lysergic acid, but with a potency much less than that of LSD. Anyone planning to take a "trip" on them will be in for an unpleasant and potentially dangerous surprise, since the seeds also contain a very unhealthy purgative resin.

PERIWINKLE, VINCA, GREATER PERIWINKLE, LESSER PERIWINKLE (*VINCA MAJOR* AND *VINCA MINOR*)

Keep these in your garden and out of your system. They contain toxic alkaloids that can cause adverse neurological actions and injure the liver and kidneys.

SPINDLE TREE (*EUONYMUS EUROPAEUS*)

An extremely violent purgative.

TONKA BEAN, TONCO BEAN, TONQUIN BEAN (*DIPTERYX ODORATA, COUMAROUNA ODORATA, DIPTERYX OPPOSITIFOLIA,* AND *COUMAROUNA OPPOSITIFOLIA*)

The active constituent of these seeds is coumarin, which the FDA prohibited marketing as a food or food additive after it was found to cause extensive liver damage, growth retardation, and testicular atrophy when used in the diet of experimental animals. (Check the labels on your OTC medicines!)

WAHOO BARK, SPINDLE TREE, EUONYMUS, BURNING BUSH (*EUONYMUS ATROPURPUREUS*)
Often used as a laxative, but though its poisonous qualities have not been thoroughly identified, it's best to play it safe and keep away from it.

WHITE SNAKEROOT, SNAKEROOT, RICHWEED (*EUPATORIUM RUGOSUM, E. OGERATOIDES,* AND *E. URTICAEFOLIUM*)
This poisonous plant contains a toxic, unsaturated alcohol. It causes "trembles" in livestock and can engender milk sickness in humans who ingest milk, butter, and possibly meat from animals who have eaten this plant.

WORMWOOD, ABSINTHIUM, ABSINTH, MADDERWORT, WERMUTH, MAGWORT, MINGWORT, WARMOT, MAGENKRAUT, HERBA ABSINTHII (*ARTEMISIA ABSINTHIUM*)
Oil of wormwood is an active narcotic poison. It is used to flavor an alcoholic liqueur—*absinthe*—which is now illegal in America because its use can damage the nervous system.

YOHIMBE (*CORYNANTHE YOHIMBI* AND *PAUSINYSTALIA YOHIMBE*)
Not an herb to play around with. It contains the toxic alkaloid yohimbine.

116. Any Questions About Chapter IX?

Does dill have any nutritive or health-giving properties?

It does indeed. It can improve appetite and digestion and also act as a diuretic. Furthermore, chewing the seeds can help eliminate bad breath.

Is it true that flaxseed is a laxative?

It can act as one. The seeds are bulk formers. Flaxseed can be eaten raw or cooked (it's great in soups), and one tablespoon daily has been found to prevent constipation in adults. It has also been found to benefit people suffering from bad coughs and bronchitis.

Are there any herbs that are okay under ordinary circumstances but might be contraindicated during pregnancy or for breast-feeding?

Well, for one, goldenseal should be avoided during pregnancy and lactation. (Berberine, the alkaloid in goldenseal, is quite similar to morphine.) Also to be avoided are caffeine-containing herbs, such as guarana and kola nuts.

Laxatives, be they natural or manufactured, should not be taken during the first few months of pregnancy, as they could cause miscarriage (buckthorn, rhubarb, and senna are natural laxatives). Strong sedative herbs like skullcap and valerian are not advisable, nor are strong spices such as capsicum and horseradish. Emetics, such as lobelia, can be dangerous early in pregnancy and in the last trimester.

Though garlic and onions are great for many things,

it might be wise to avoid them if you're either pregnant or nursing, especially during the latter, as they have been known to pass through the breast milk and produce colic in infants.

X

How to Find Out What Vitamins You Really Need

117. What Is a Balanced Diet and Are You Eating It?

A balanced diet is something easily found in books and rarely on the table. Though nutrients are widely scattered all through our food supply, soil depletion, storage, food processing, and cooking destroy many of them. Still, there are enough left to make balancing meals important. After all, supplements cannot work without food, and the better the food you eat, the more effective your supplements will be. Unfortunately, no possible "balanced" diet is likely to meet nutritional needs today.

Nevertheless, to know whether or not you are balancing your meals, you should become familiar with the four basic food groups, and the recommended number of portions that should be eaten from them each day. Serving sizes should be individually determined; smaller amounts for less active people, larger amounts for teenagers and people who do physically strenuous work.

MILK GROUP

Milk, cheese, yogurt, foods made from milk.

    3 servings per day for a child
    4 servings per day for a teenager
    2 servings per day for an adult
    4 servings per day for pregnant and
        lactating women

MEAT GROUP

Beef, veal, pork, lamb, fish, poultry, liver, or eggs.
Dry peas, beans, soy extenders, and nuts combined
with animal protein—including eggs, milk, and cheese—
or grain protein can be substituted for meat serving.

    2 servings per day
    3 servings per day for pregnant women

FRUIT-VEGETABLE GROUP

Citrus or other fruit rich in vitamin C (or tomato
juice) should be eaten daily. Dark green, leafy, or
orange vegetables and fruit should be eaten three or four
times a week for vitamin A.

    4 servings per day

GRAIN GROUP

Whole or enriched grains, bread in any shape, hot or
cold cereals, macaroni, noodles, or other pasta.

    4 servings per day

The recommended servings, as outined by the National
Research Council, are designed to supply 1,200 calories.

You are expected to adjust the size of the servings to suit your own individual growth, weight, and energy needs.

118. How to Test for Deficiencies

If you're wondering whether or not you need vitamin or mineral supplementation, your best bet would be to contact a nutritionally oriented doctor (see section 278). Other than that, there are a variety of "indicator" tests that should tell you enough to point you in the right supplement direction.

Dr. John M. Ellis has devised a quick early-warning test for B_6 (pyridoxine) deficiency. Extend your hand, palm up, then try to bend the two joints in your four fingers (not the knuckles of your hand) until your fingertips reach your palm. (This is not a fist, only two joints are bent.) Do this with both hands. If it is difficult, if finger joints don't allow tips to reach your palm, a pyridoxine deficiency is likely.

Betty Lee Morales, a well-known nutritionist, says that urine is a fair indicator of B vitamin concentration in your body. Since B vitamins are water soluble and lost each day through excretion, when your body demands more your urine will often be light in color. When the urine is dark, your B demands are most likely less. (Caution: Many drugs, illnesses—particularly hepatitis—and foods also alter urine color. This should be taken into consideration and checked with your doctor.)

Hair analyses, where a tablespoon of hair clipped from the back of the neck is sent to the laboratory to check for deficient or abnormally high mineral levels, have recently become a subject of controversy regarding their reliability. Hair analysts say that hair can serve as a permanent record of nutrition consumption and toxic exposure, since substances entering the hair stay there until the hair falls out. Their detractors, on the other hand, say that there are too many factors besides what we eat and drink that can influence the content of hair (dyes, shampoos, colorings, waving lotions, pool chemicals, and so on) to provide a reliable analysis.

As of this writing, the controversy has not been resolved either way. So my advice, once again, is to check with a nutritionally oriented doctor before investing in an analysis on your own.

Probably the best indicator of any vitamin or mineral deficiency is your body—and the way that it's feeling.

119. Possible Warning Signs

A body in need of vitamins usually lets you know about it sooner or later. It's unlikely that any of us will come down with scurvy before realizing we need vitamin C, but more often than not our bodies are giving us clues that we just don't recognize. With the price of medical insurance rising daily, paying attention to your nutritional warning system is about the best and cheapest insurance around. Here are a few common symptoms that you might be ignoring—and shouldn't.

The supplements recommended are not intended as medical advice, only as a guide in working with your doctor.

NOTE: MVP stands for Mindell Vitamin Program (or Most Valuable Player in the nutrition game). It consists of a high-potency multiple vitamin with chelated minerals, preferably time release; a vitamin C, 1,000 mg.

with bioflavonoids, rutin, hesperidin, and rose hips, time release; and a high-potency chelated multiple-mineral supplement.

POSSIBLE DEFICIENCY	ARE YOU EATING ENOUGH?

SYMPTOM: Appetite Loss

Protein	Meat, fish, eggs, dairy products, soybeans, peanuts
Vitamin A	Fish, liver, egg yolks, butter, cream, green leafy or yellow vegetables
Vitamin B$_1$	Brewer's yeast, whole grains, meat (pork or liver), nuts, legumes, potatoes
Vitamin C	Citrus fruits, tomatoes, potatoes, cabbage, green peppers
Biotin	Brewer's yeast, nuts, beef liver, kidney, unpolished rice
Phosphorus	Milk, cheese, meat, poultry, fish, cereals, nuts legumes
Sodium	Beef, pork, sardines, cheese, green olives, corn bread, sauerkraut
Zinc	Vegetables, whole grains, wheat bran, wheat germ, pumpkin seeds, sunflower seeds

RECOMMENDED SUPPLEMENT: 1 B complex, 50 mg., taken with each meal
  1 B$_{12}$ 2,000 mcg. (time release) with breakfast
  1 organic iron complex tablet (containing vitamin C, copper, liver, manganese, and zinc to help assimilate iron)

SYMPTOM: Bad Breath

Niacin	Liver, meat, fish, whole grains, legumes

RECOMMENDED SUPPLEMENT: 1–2 tbsp. acidophilus liquid (flavored) 1–3 times daily
  1 chlorophyll tablet or capsule 3 times daily
  1–3 chelated zinc 50-mg. tabs. 3 times daily
  1–2 multiple digestive enzyme tabs. 1–3 times daily

POSSIBLE DEFICIENCY   ARE YOU EATING ENOUGH?

SYMPTOM: *Body Odor*

B_{12} Yeast, liver, beef, eggs, kidney
Zinc   Vegetables, whole grains, wheat bran, wheat
                           germ, pumpkin seeds, sunflower seeds

RECOMMENDED SUPPLEMENT: 1–2 tbsp. acidophilus liquid (flavored) 1–3
                               times daily
                           1 chlorophyll tablet or capsule 3 times daily
                           1–3 chelated zinc tabs., 15–50 mg. 3 times
                               daily
                           1–2 multiple digestive enzyme tabs. 1–3 times
                               daily

SYMPTOM: *Bruising Easily* (when slight or minor injuries produce
bluish, purplish discoloration of skin)

Vitamin C   Citrus fruits, tomatoes, potatoes, cabbage, green
                           peppers
Bioflavonoids   Orange, lemon, lime, tangerine peels

RECOMMENDED SUPPLEMENT: 1 C complex, 1,000 mg. (time release) with
                           bioflavonoids, rutin, and hesperidin A.M. and
                           P.M.

SYMPTOM: *High Cholesterol*

B complex   Yeast, brewer's yeast, dried lima beans, raisins,
Inositol   cantaloupe

RECOMMENDED SUPPLEMENT: 2 tbsp. lecithin granules 3 times daily (used
                               on salads or on cottage cheese)
                           or
                           3 1,200-mg. caps lecithin 3–4 times daily

POSSIBLE DEFICIENCY	ARE YOU EATING ENOUGH?

SYMPTOM: *Constipation*

B complex	Liver, beef, cheese, pork, kidney

RECOMMENDED SUPPLEMENT: 8–10 glasses of water daily
1 tbsp. acidophilus liquid 3 times daily
3–9 bran tabs. daily or 3 tbsp. bran daily

SYMPTOM: *Diarrhea*

Vitamin K	Yogurt, alfalfa, soybean oil, fish-liver oils, kelp
Niacin	Liver, lean meat, brewer's yeast, wheat germ, peanuts, dried nutritional yeast, white meat of poultry, avocado, fish, legumes, whole grain
Vitamin F	Vegetable oils, peanuts, sunflower seeds, walnuts

RECOMMENDED SUPPLEMENT: 1 g. potassium divided over 3 meals
As a preventive 1–2 tbsp. acidophilus liquid
(flavored) 3 times daily

SYMPTOM: *Dizziness*

Manganese	Nuts, green leafy vegetables, peas, beets, egg yolks
B₂ (riboflavin)	Milk, liver, kidney, yeast, cheese, fish, eggs

RECOMMENDED SUPPLEMENT: 50–100 mg. niacin 3 times a day
400 IU vitamin E 1–3 times a day

SYMPTOM: *Ear Noises*

Manganese	Nuts, green leafy vegetables, peas, beets, egg yolks
Potassium	Bananas, watercress, all leafy green vegetables, citrus fruits, sunflower seeds

RECOMMENDED SUPPLEMENT: 50-100 mg. niacin 3 times a day
400 IU vitamin E1–3 times a day

POSSIBLE DEFICIENCY   ARE YOU EATING ENOUGH?

SYMPTOM: *Eye Problems* (night blindness, inability to adjust to darkness, bloodshot eyes, inflammations, burning sensations, sties)

Vitamin A	Fish, liver, egg yolks, butter, cream, green leafy or yellow vegetables
B₂ (riboflavin)	Milk, liver, kidney, yeast, cheese, fish, eggs

RECOMMENDED SUPPLEMENT: 10,000 IU vitamin A 1–3 times daily for 5 days and stop for 2

100 mg. B complex (time release), 1 in A.M. and P.M.

500 mg. vitamin C with bioflavonoids, rutin, and hesperidin, 1 in A.M. and P.M.

400 IU vitamin E (dry), 1 in A.M. and P.M.

SYMPTOM: *Fatigue* (lassitude, weakness, no inclination for physical activity)

Zinc	Vegetables, whole-grain products, brewer's yeast, wheat bran, wheat germ, pumpkin and sunflower seeds
Carbohydrates	Cellulose
Protein	Meat, fish, eggs, dairy products, soybeans, peanuts
Vitamin A	Fish, liver, egg yolks, butter, cream, green leafy or yellow vegetables
Vitamin B complex PABA	Yeast, brewer's yeast, dried lima beans, raisins, cantaloupe
Iron	Wheat germ, soybean flour, beef, kidney, liver, beans, clams, peaches, molasses
Iodine	Seafoods, dairy products, kelp
Vitamin C	Citrus fruits, tomatoes, potatoes, cabbage, green peppers
Vitamin D	Fish-liver oils, butter, egg yolks, liver, sunshine

RECOMMENDED SUPPLEMENT: 1 B complex, 100 mg. (time release), 2 times daily

1 2,000 mcg. B₁₂ A.M. and P.M.

MVP, 1 A.M. and P.M.

SYMPTOM: *Gastrointestinal Problems* (gastritis, gastric ulcers, gallbladder, digestive disturbances)

Vitamin B₁ (thiamine)	Brewer's yeast, whole grains, meat (pork or liver), nuts, legumes, potatoes
Vitamin B₂ (riboflavin)	Milk, liver, kidney, yeast, cheese, fish, eggs
Folic acid (folacin)	Fresh green leafy vegetables, fruit, organ meats, liver, dried nutritional yeast
PABA	Yeast, brewer's yeast, dried lima beans, raisins, cantaloupe
Vitamin C	Citrus fruits, tomatoes, potatoes, cabbage, green peppers
Chlorine	Kelp, rye flour, ripe olives, sea greens
Pantothenic acid	Yeast, brewer's yeast, dried lima beans, raisins, cantaloupe

RECOMMENDED SUPPLEMENT: 10,000 IU vitamin A, 1–2 times daily; take for 5 days and stop for 2

100 mg. B complex (time release), 1 A.M. and P.M.

Multiple minerals, 1 A.M. and P.M.

Betaine HCl 500 mg. ½ hour before meals with glass of water

Multiple digestive enzyme ½ hour after meals with glass of water

Fresh-squeezed cabbage juice, 1 glass after meals

SYMPTOM: *Hair Problems*

1. DANDRUFF (loose flakes—dry or yellow and greasy—which fall from scalp)

Vitamin B₁₂ (cyanocobalamin)	Liver, beef, pork, organ meats, eggs, milk and milk products
Vitamin F	Vegetable oils, peanuts, sunflower seeds, walnuts
Vitamin B₆	Dried nutritional yeast, liver, organ meats, legumes, whole-grain cereals, fish
Selenium	Bran, germ of cereals, broccoli, onions, tomatoes, tuna

RECOMMENDED SUPPLEMENT: 100 mcg. selenium twice daily

1 MVP A.M. and P.M.

3 vitamin F caps 3 times daily with meals

POSSIBLE DEFICIENCY   ARE YOU EATING ENOUGH?

---

2. DULL, DRY, BRITTLE, OR GRAYING HAIR

Vitamin B complex   Yeast, brewer's yeast, dried, lima beans, raisins,
PABA   cantaloupe
Vitamin F   Vegetable oils, peanuts, sunflower seeds,
                           walnuts
Iodine   Seafood, iodized salt, dairy products

RECOMMENDED SUPPLEMENT: 3 vitamin F caps with each meal
                           3–6 lecithin caps with each meal
                           1 MVP A.M. and P.M.

---

3. LOSS OF HAIR

Biotin   Brewer's yeast, nuts, beef liver, kidney,
                           unpolished rice
Inositol   Unrefined molasses and liver, lecithin,
                           unprocessed whole grains, citrus fruits, brewer's
                           yeast
Chlorine   Sodium chloride (table salt)
B complex with C   Yeast, brewer's yeast, dried lima beans, raisins,
and folic acid   cantaloupe, citrus fruits, green peppers, tomatoes,
                           cabbage, potatoes, fresh green leafy vegetables,
                           fruit, organ meats, liver, dried nutritional yeast

RECOMMENDED SUPPLEMENT: 1,000 mg. choline and inositol daily
                           1 multiple mineral daily
                           Cysteine 1 g. daily
                           Vitamin C 3,000 mg. daily
                           B complex 100 mg. (time release) A.M. and
                           P.M.

SYMPTOM: *Heart Palpitation*

Vitamin B$_{12}$ Yeast, liver, beef, eggs, kidney
(cobalamin,
cyanocobalamin)

RECOMMENDED SUPPLEMENT: 1 MVP A.M. and P.M.
                           100 mg. vitamin B complex (time release)
                              A.M. and P.M.
                           100 mg. niacin 1–3 times daily
                           3 caps lecithin 3 times daily

POSSIBLE DEFICIENCY   ARE YOU EATING ENOUGH?

SYMPTOM: *High Blood Pressure*

Choline   Egg yolks, brain, heart, green leafy vegetables, yeast, liver, wheat germ

RECOMMENDED SUPPLEMENT: Lecithin granules, 3 tbsp. daily or 3 caps 3 times daily
                          1 MVP A.M. and P.M.
                          Start with 100 IU vitamin E and work up to higher strengths. (See section 39.)
                          1–3 kelp tabs. daily
                          1 garlic perle 3 times daily

SYMPTOM: *Infections*
(high susceptibility)

Vitamin A   Fish, liver, egg yolks, butter, cream, green
(carotene)   leafy or yellow vegetables
Pantothenic acid   Yeast, brewer's yeast, dried lima beans, raisins, cantaloupe

RECOMMENDED SUPPLEMENT: 1–2 tbsp. acidophilus 3 times daily
                          Vitamin A up to 100,000 IU every other day for duration of infection
                          1 MVP A.M. and P.M. (2–5 g. vitamin C for duration of infection)

SYMPTOM: *Insomnia*

Potassium   Bananas, watercress, all leafy green vegetables, citrus fruits, sunflower seeds
B complex   Yeast, brewer's yeast, dried lima beans, raisins, cantaloupe
Biotin   Brewer's yeast, nuts, beef liver, kidney, unpolished rice
Calcium   Milk and milk products, meat, fish, eggs, cereal products, beans, fruit, vegetables

RECOMMENDED SUPPLEMENT: 2 g. tryptophan ½ hr. before bedtime (see section 76)
                          Vitamin B_6 100 mg., niacinamide 100 mg., niacinamide 100 mg., and chelated calcium and magnesium ½ hr. before bedtime
                          1 MVP A.M. and P.M.

POSSIBLE DEFICIENCY   ARE YOU EATING ENOUGH?

SYMPTOM: *Loss of Smell*

Vitamin A   Fish, liver, egg yolks, butter, cream, green
                         leafy or yellow vegetables
Zinc   Vegetables, whole grains, wheat bran, wheat
                         germ, pumpkin and sunflower seeds

RECOMMENDED SUPPLEMENT: 50 mg. chelated zinc 3 times daily (cut back
                         to 1–2 daily when condition improves)

SYMPTOM: *Memory Loss*

B₁ (thiamine)   Brewer's yeast, whole grains, meat (pork or
                         liver), nuts, legumes, potatoes

RECOMMENDED SUPPLEMENT: L-glutamine, 500 mg. 3 times daily
                         50 mg. B complex A.M. and P.M.
                         Choline, 2 g. daily in divided doses

---

SYMPTOM: *Menstrual Problems*

B₁₂   Yeast, liver, beef, eggs, kidney

RECOMMENDED SUPPLEMENT: 7–10 days before period:
                         1 MVP A.M. and P.M.
                         100 mg. B₆ 3 times daily
                         100 mg. B complex (time release) A.M. and
                         P.M.
                         Evening primrose oil, 500 mg. 3 times daily
                         500 mg. magnesium and ½ as much calcium
                         once daily

SYMPTOM: *Mouth Sores and Cracks*

Vitamin B₂ (riboflavin) Milk, liver, kidney, yeast, cheese, fish, eggs
Vitamin B₆ (pyridoxine) Dried nutritional yeast, liver, organ meats,
                         legumes, whole-grain cereals, fish

RECOMMENDED SUPPLEMENT: 50 mg. B complex 3 times daily with meals
                         1 MVP A.M. and P.M.

POSSIBLE DEFICIENCY   ARE YOU EATING ENOUGH?

SYMPTOM: *Muscle Cramps* (general muscle weakness, tenderness in calf, night cramps, charley horse)

Vitamin B_1 (thiamine)	Brewer's yeast, whole grains, meat (pork or liver), nuts, legumes, potatoes
Vitamin B_6 (pyridoxine)	Dried nutritional yeast, liver, organ meats, legumes, whole-grain cereals, fish
Biotin	Brewer's yeast, nuts, beef liver, kidney, unpolished rice
Chlorine	Sodium chloride (table salt)
Sodium	Beef, pork, sardines, cheese, green olives, corn bread, sauerkraut
Vitamin D (calciferol)	Fish-liver oils, butter, egg yolks, liver, sunshine

RECOMMENDED SUPPLEMENT: 400 IU vitamin E (dry) 3 times daily
                           Chelated calcium and magnesium, 3 tabs 3 times daily
                           100 mg. niacin 3 times daily

SYMPTOM: *Nervousness*

Vitamin B_6 (pyridoxine)	Dried nutritional yeast, liver, organ meats, legumes, whole-grain cereals, fish
Vitamin B_{12} (cyanocobalamin)	Yeast, liver, beef, eggs, kidney
Niacin (nicotinic acid, niacinamide)	Liver, meat, fish, whole grains, legumes
PABA	Yeast, brewer's yeast, dried lima beans, raisins, cantaloupe
Magnesium	Green leafy vegetables, nuts, cereals, grains, seafood

RECOMMENDED SUPPLEMENT: Stress B with C 1–3 times daily (50 mg. of all B vitamins)
                           500–667 mg. tryptophan 3 times daily between meals (with juice or water) and 3 tabs at bedtime
                           3 chelated calcium and magnesium tabs 3 times daily
                           1 MVP A.M. and P.M.

POSSIBLE DEFICIENCY   ARE YOU EATING ENOUGH?

SYMPTOM: *Nosebleeds*

Vitamin C	Citrus fruits, tomatoes, potatoes, cabbage, green peppers
Vitamin K	Yogurt, alfalfa, soybean oil, fish-liver oils, kelp
Bioflavonoids	Orange, lemon, lime, tangerine peels

RECOMMENDED SUPPLEMENT: 1,000 mg. vitamin C with 50 mg. rutin, hesperidin, and 500 mg. bioflavonoids (time release) A.M. and P.M.

SYMPTOM: *Retarded Growth*

Fat	Meat, butter
Protein	Meat, fish, eggs, dairy products, soybeans, peanuts
Vitamin B$_2$ (riboflavin)	Milk, liver, kidney, yeast, cheese, fish, eggs
Folic acid	Fresh green leafy vegetables, fruit, organ meats, liver, dried nutritional yeast
Zinc	Vegetables, whole grains, wheat bran, wheat germ, pumpkin and sunflower seeds
Cobalt	Liver, kidney, pancreas, and spleen (organ meats)

RECOMMENDED SUPPLEMENT: 1 MVP A.M. and P.M.

SYMPTOM: *Skin Problems*

1. ACNE (face blemishes, thickened skin, blackheads, whiteheads, red spots)

Water-solubilized vitamin A	Fish, liver, egg yolks, butter, cream, green leafy or yellow vegetables
Vitamin B complex	Yeast, brewer's yeast, dried lima beans, raisins, cantaloupe

RECOMMENDED SUPPLEMENT: 1 multiple vitamin-mineral (low in iodine) daily
1–2 400 IU vitamin E (dry) daily
25,000 IU vitamin A (dry), 1–2 tabs. daily 5 days a week
50 mg. chelated zinc 3 times daily with food
1–2 tbsp. acidophilus liquid 3 times daily or 3–6 caps 3 times daily
(Iodine worsens acne, so eliminate all processed foods—high in iodized salt—from your diet)

POSSIBLE DEFICIENCY	ARE YOU EATING ENOUGH?

2. DERMATITIS
(skin inflammation)

Vitamin B$_2$ (riboflavin)	Milk, liver, kidney, yeast, cheese, fish, eggs
Vitamin B$_6$ (pyridoxine)	Dried nutritional yeast, liver, organ meats, legumes, whole-grain cereals, fish
Biotin	Brewer's yeast, nuts, beef liver, kidney, unpolished rice
Niacin (nicotinic acid, niacinamide)	Liver, meat, fish, whole grains, legumes

RECOMMENDED SUPPLEMENT:
1 multiple vitamin-mineral (low in iodine) daily
1–2 400 IU vitamin E (dry) daily
25,000 IU vitamin A (dry), 1–2 tabs. daily 5 days a week
50 mg. chelated zinc 3 times daily with food
1–2 tbsp. acidophilus liquid 3 times daily or 3–6 caps 3 times daily

---

3. ECZEMA (rough, dry, scaly skin, redness and swelling, small blisters)

Fat	Meat, butter
Vitamin A (carotene)	Fish, liver, egg yolks, butter, cream, green leafy or yellow vegetables
Vitamin B complex Inositol	Yeast, brewer's yeast, dried lima beans, raisins, cantaloupe
Copper	Organ meats, oysters, nuts, dried legumes, whole-grain cereals
Iodine	Seafood, iodized salt, dairy products

RECOMMENDED SUPPLEMENT:
1 multiple vitamin-mineral (low in iodine) daily
1–2 400 IU vitamin E (dry) daily
25,000 IU vitamin A (dry), 1–2 tabs. daily 5 days a week
50 mg. chelated zinc 3 times daily with food
1–2 tbsp. acidophilus liquid 3 times daily or 3–6 caps 3 times daily

---

SYMPTOM: *Slow-Healing Wounds and Fractures*

Vitamin C	Citrus fruits, tomatoes, potatoes, cabbage, green peppers

RECOMMENDED SUPPLEMENT:
50 mg. zinc 3 times daily
400 IU vitamin E 3 times daily
1 MVP A.M. and P.M.

POSSIBLE DEFICIENCY   ARE YOU EATING ENOUGH?

SYMPTOM: *Softening of Bones and Teeth*

Vitamin D (calciferol)   Fish-liver oils, butter, egg yolks, liver, sunshine
Calcium   Milk and milk products, meat, fish, eggs, cereal
                               products, beans, fruit, vegetables

RECOMMENDED SUPPLEMENT: 1,000–1,500 mg. calcium, 500 mg. magnesium
                               divided over 2 meals daily

SYMPTOM: *Tremors*

Magnesium   Green leafy vegetables, nuts, cereals, grains,
                               seafood

RECOMMENDED SUPPLEMENT: B complex and 50 mg. B_6 3 times daily
                               1,000 mg. calcium, 500 mg. magnesium
                               divided over 3 meals daily

SYMPTOM: *Vaginal Itching*

Vitamin B_2 Milk, liver, kidney, yeast, cheese, fish, eggs

RECOMMENDED SUPPLEMENT: 2 tbsp. acidophilus 3 times daily or 3–6 caps
                               3–4 times daily
                               (Acidophilus or vinegar douche can also help.)

SYMPTOM: *Water Retention*

Vitamin B_6 Dried nutritional yeast, liver, organ meats,
                               legumes, whole-grain cereals, fish

RECOMMENDED SUPPLEMENT: 100 mg. B_6 3 times daily

SYMPTOM: *White Spots on Nails*

Zinc   Vegetables, whole grains, wheat bran, wheat
                               germ, pumpkin and sunflower seeds

RECOMMENDED SUPPLEMENT: 50 mg. zinc 3 times daily
                               Stress B with C 1–2 times daily
                               1 multiple mineral 2 times daily

120. Cravings—What They Might Mean

Cravings, which can sometimes mean allergies, are more often nature's way of letting you know that you're not getting enough of certain vitamins or minerals. Frequently these specific hungers develop because overall diet is inadequate.

Some of the most common cravings are:

Peanut butter   This is definitely among the top ten, and it's not at all surprising. Peanut butter is a rich source of B vitamins. If you find yourself dipping into the jar often, it might be because you're under stress and your ordinary B intake has become insufficient. Since 50 g. of peanut butter—a third of a cup—is 284 calories, you'll find it easier on your waistline to take a B-complex supplement if you do not want to gain weight.

Bananas   When you catch yourself reaching for this fruit again and again, it could be because your body needs potassium. One medium banana has 555 mg. People taking diuretics or cortisone (which rob the body of needed potassium) often crave bananas.

Cheese   If you're more a cheese luster than a cheese lover, there's a good chance that your real hunger is for calcium and phosphorus. (If it's processed cheese that you've been snacking on, you've been getting aluminum and salt, too, without knowing it.) For one thing, you might try eating more broccoli. That's high in calcium and phosphorus, and a lot lower in calories than cheese.

Apples   An apple a day doesn't necessarily keep the doctor away, but it offers a lot of good things that you might be missing in other foods—calcium, magnesium, phosphorus, potassium—and is an excellent source of cholesterol-lowering pectin! If you have a tendency to eat a lot of saturated fat, it could account for your apple cravings.

Butter Most often vegetarians crave butter because of their own low-saturated-fat intake. Salted butter, on the other hand, might be craved for the salt alone.

Cola The craving for cola is most often a sugar hunger and an addiction to caffeine. (See section 229.) The beverage has no nutritive value.

Nuts If you're a little nutty about nuts, you probably could use more protein, B vitamins, or fat in your diet. If it's salted nuts you favor, you could be craving the sodium and not the nuts. You'll find that people under stress tend to eat more nuts than relaxed individuals.

Ice cream High as ice cream is in calcium, most people crave it for its sugar content. Hypoglycemics and diabetics have great hungers for it, as do people seeking to recapture the security of childhood.

Pickles If you're pregnant and want pickles, you're probably after the salt. And if you're not pregnant and crave pickles, the reason is most likely the same. (Pickles also contain a substantial amount of potassium.)

Bacon Cravings for bacon are usually because of its fat. People on restricted diets are most susceptible to greasy binges. Unfortunately, saturated fat is not bacon's only drawback. Bacon is very high in carcinogenic nitrites. If you do indulge in bacon, be sure you're ingesting enough of vitamins C and A, D, and E to counteract the nitrites.

Eggs Aside from the protein (two eggs give you 13 g.), sulfur, amino acids, and selenium protein, egg lovers might also be seeking the yolk's fat content or, paradoxically, its cholesterol-and-fat-dissolving choline.

Cantaloupe   Just because you like its taste might not be the only reason you crave this melon. Cantaloupe is high in potassium and vitamin A. In fact, a quarter of a melon has 3,400 IU vitamin A. Since the melon also offers vitamin C, calcium, magnesium, phosphorus, biotin, and inositol, it's not a bad craving to give in to. There're only about sixty calories in half a melon.

Olives   Whether you crave them green or black, you're likely to be after the salt. People with underactive thyroids are most often the first to reach for them.

Salt   No guesswork here, it's the sodium you're after. Cravers quite possibly have a thyroid iodine deficiency or low-sodium Addison's disease. Hypertensives often crave salt, and shouldn't.

Onions   Cravings for spicy foods can sometimes indicate problems in the lungs or sinuses.

Chocolate   Definitely one of the foremost cravings, if not *the* foremost. Chocoholics are addicted to the caffeine as well as the sugar (there are 5 to 10 mg. of caffeine in a cup of cocoa). If you want to kick the chocolate habit, try carob instead. (Carob, also called St. John's bread, is made from the edible pods of the Mediterranean carob tree.)

Milk   If you're still craving milk as an adult, you might need a calcium supplement. Then again, it might be the amino acids—such as tryptophan, leucine, and lysine—that your body needs. Nervous people often seek out the tryptophan in milk, since it has a very soothing effect.

Chinese food   Of course it's delicious, but often it's the monosodium glutamate in the food that fosters the craving. People with salt deficiencies usually go all out for Chinese food. (MSG can cause a histamine reaction in some individuals. Headaches and flushing may occur.

Most Chinese restaurants will now prepare your food without MSG if you request it.)

Mayonnaise Since this is a fatty food, it is often craved by vegetarians and people who have eliminated other fats from their diet.

Tart fruits A persistent craving for tart fruits can often indicate problems with the gallbladder or liver.

Paint and dirt Children have a tendency to eat paint and dirt. Frequently this is an indication of a calcium or vitamin-D deficiency. A hard reevaluation of your child's diet is essential, and a visit to your pediatrician is recommended.

121. Getting the Most Vitamins from Your Food

Eating the right foods doesn't necessarily mean that you're getting the vitamins they contain. Food processing, storing, and cooking can easily undermine the best nutritious intentions. To get the most from what you eat (not to mention what you spend) keep the following tips in mind.

• Wash but don't soak fresh vegetables if you hope to benefit from the B vitamins and C they contain.

• Forgo convenience and make your salads when you're ready to eat them. Fruits and vegetables cut up and left to stand lose vitamins.

• Use a sharp knife when cutting or shredding fresh vegetables, because vitamins A and C are diminished when vegetable tissues are bruised.

• If you don't plan to eat your fresh fruit or vegetables for a few days, you're better off buying flash-frozen ones. The vitamin content of good frozen green beans will be higher than those fresh ones you've kept in your refrigerator for a week.

• Outer green leaves of lettuce, though coarser than inner ones, have higher calcium, iron, and vitamin A content.

• Don't thaw your frozen vegetables before cooking.

• Broccoli leaves have a higher vitamin A value than the flower buds or stalks.

• There are more vitamins in converted and parboiled rice than in polished rice, and brown rice is more nutritious than white.

• Frozen foods that you can boil in their bags offer more vitamins than the ordinary kind, and all frozen foods are preferable to canned ones.

• Cooking in copper pots can destroy vitamin C, folic acid, and vitamin E.

• Stainless steel, glass, and enamel are the best utensils for retaining nutrients while cooking. (Iron pots can give you the benefit of that mineral, but they will shortchange you on vitamin C.)

• The shortest cooking time and the smallest amount of water are the least destructive to nutrients.

• Milk in glass containers can lose riboflavin, as well as vitamins A and D, unless kept out of the light. (Breads exposed to light can also lose these nutrients.)

• Well-browned, crusty, or toasted baked goods have less thiamine than others.

• Bake and boil potatoes in their skins to get the most vitamins from them.

• Use cooking water from vegetables to make soups, juices from meats for gravies, and syrups from canned fruits to make desserts.

• Refrain from using any baking soda when cooking

vegetables if you want to benefit from their thiamine and vitamin C.
• Store vegetables and fruits in the refrigerator as soon as you bring them home from the market.

122. Any Questions About Chapter X?

I feed my children what I think is a pretty well balanced diet. But they're teenagers and when they're out they often have burgers, hot dogs, shakes, and that sort of junk food. Are these really bad for them?

Well, ounce for ounce, munch for munch, and sip for sip, the bad outweighs the good. For instance, a fast-food burger can supply 44 percent of a teenage boy's requirement for protein. But when you consider that a Big Mac, for example, is also supplying 591 calories, 33 grams of fat, 6 *grams* of sugar, and 963 mg. of sodium (a Burger King Whopper has *1,083 mg. of sodium*), you have to admit that's an awfully high nutritional price to pay for protein. No one needs .all that salt (see section 256).

As for hot dogs, there's very little good to say about them. They're a high-fat, low-protein meat and usually contain sodium or potassium nitrite. Nitrites combine with substances called amines, commonly found in foods, and form nitrosamines, which have been found to be carcinogenic (cancer-causing).

Shakes, which do contain milk or a milk product, also contain 8 to 14 teaspoons of sugar and 276 to 685 mg. of salt. Your kids could blend one up at home for half the price, calories, sugar, and salt—and double the nutritional value. Passing this information along to your children might be a good way to get them to pass up those fast-food places.

Very often I experience a sort of hot, burning feeling on my tongue and lips. It doesn't seem to be related to any foods I've eaten. Could it indicate a vitamin deficiency?

It's very possible. The feeling of having a burning tongue or lips has in many instances been linked to a vitamin B_1 (thiamine) deficiency. I'd suggest increasing your intake of whole wheat, oatmeal, bran, vegetables, and brewer's yeast, along with taking a balanced vitamin B complex, 100 mg., 3 times a day.

My mother has a craving for ice. Not just on hot days, but all the time. She chews cubes as if they were candy. Could this sort of craving have anything to do with a dietary deficiency?

If your mother is often tired, her craving for ice might indicate an iron deficiency (which can cause a low-grade anemia). You might try encouraging her to add more iron-rich foods to her diet (liver, dried peaches, red meat, oysters, asparagus, oatmeal) and to take an organic iron supplement, 50–100 mg., 1 to 3 times a day.

I'm forty-two years old and am developing yellowish growths around my eyes. Is there some vitamin or nutrient that's missing from my diet that could be causing this?

More likely those growths are cholesterol deposits, which can occur when the body is trying to rid itself of excess cholesterol. This sort of condition tends to run in families and could possibly indicate that you're in the high-risk heart disease percentile. See section 87 for how to reduce cholesterol. Also, increase your intake of vitamin B, chromium, and zinc, in foods and supplements.

XI

Read the Label

123. The Importance of Understanding What's on Labels

All too often people buy supplements and never even look at the labels. They ask a clerk for a multivitamin and take what they are given, not realizing that they might be getting shortchanged on the vitamin content. All multivitamins differ in amounts included, and the most expensive tablet is not necessarily the best. The only way to be sure you're getting the B_6, folacin, or C that you need is to read the small print on the label. Also, if you have any allergies, it's wise to check what else you're getting with your supplement. (See section 21.)

If there are words on the label that you don't understand, ask the pharmacist or vitamin clerk to explain them. If they can't, buy your supplements where someone can. And above all, remember to check the dosage you're getting. If you've been instructed to take vitamin E four times a day, it's unlikely that you want 400 IU. Vitamins and minerals come in different strengths. Be sure you're getting what you ask for—and need. Not understanding labels can often negate a lot of vitamin benefits.

124. How Does That Measure Up?

> IU, RE, MG, MCG—a little
> can mean a lot.

The terminology for measuring vitamin activity is not as confusing as you might think. Fat-soluble vitamins (A, E, D, and K) are usually measured in international units (IU). Recently, though, an expert committee of the Food and Agriculture Organization/World Health Organization (FAO/WHO) decided to change this order of measurement for vitamin A. Instead of using international units, they proposed that vitamin A be evaluated in terms of retinol equivalents (RE), that is, the equivalent weight of retinol (vitamin A_1, alcohol) *actually absorbed and converted*.

Retinol equivalents come out to about five times less than international units (IU). Recommended allowances of 5,000 IU for a male between the ages of twenty-three and fifty would only be 1,000 RE; 4,000 IU for similarly aged females would only be 800 RE.

Most other vitamins and minerals are measured in milligrams (mg.) and micrograms (mcg.). If you know that 1 g. equals 0.35 ounce, that it takes 28.35 g. to equal 1 ounce (and 1 fluid ounce equals 2 tablespoons), you'll have a better idea of just how much—or rather, how little—it takes for vitamins and minerals to do their job. The following table is a handy guide to refer to:

WHAT'S WHAT IN WEIGHTS AND MEASURES

Metric Measure

1 kilogram equals 1,000 grams
1 gram equal 1,000 milligrams

1 milligram equals 1/1,000th part of a gram
1 microgram equals 1/1,000th part of a milligram
1 gamma equals 1 microgram

Avoirdupois Weight

16 ounces equal 1 pound
7,000 grains equal 1 pound
453.6 grams equal 1 pound
1 ounce av. equals 437.5 grains
1 ounce av. equals 28.35 grams

Conversion Factors

1 gram equals 15.4 grains
1 grain equals 0.065 grams (65 milligrams)
1 ounce apothecary equals 31.1 grams
1 fluid ounce equals 29.8 cc.
1 fluid ounce equals 480 minims

Liquid Measure

1 drop equals 1 minim
1 minim equals 0.06 cc.
15 minims equal 1.0 cc.
4 cc. equal 1 fluid dram
30 cc. equal 1 fluid ounce

Household Measure

1 teaspoon equals 4 cc. equals 1 fluid gram
1 tablespoon equals 15 cc. equals ½ fluid ounce
½ pint equals 240 cc. equals 8 fluid ounces

Abbreviations

AMDR	Adult Minimum Daily Requirement
USP Unit	United States Pharmocopeia
IU	International Unit

MDR	Minimum Daily Requirement
mg.	milligram
mcg.	microgram
g.	gram
gr.	grain

125. Breaking the RDA Code

Many people are bewildered by the variances between vitamin standards listed as RDA, U.S. RDA, and MDR. It becomes much less confusing when you understand that they are not the same thing.

RDA (Recommended Daily Dietary Allowances) came into being in 1941, when the Food and Nutrition Board of the National Research Council of the Academy of Sciences was established by the government to safeguard public health. The RDA are not formulated to cover the needs of those who are ill—they are not therapeutic and are meant strictly for healthy individuals— nor do they take into account nutrient losses that occur during processing and preparation. They are *estimates* of nutritional needs necessary to ensure satisfactory growth of children and the prevention of nutrient depletion in adults. *They are not meant to be optimal intakes, nor are they recommendations for an ideal diet.* They are not average requirements but recommendations intended to meet the needs of those *healthy* people with the highest requirements.

U.S. RDA (U.S. Recommended Daily Allowances) were formulated by the Food and Drug Administration (FDA) to be used as the *legal* standards for food labeling in regard to nutrient content. (The RDA were used as the basis for the U.S. RDA.) Calories and ten nutrients must be listed on food labels—protein, carbohydrate, fat, vitamin A, vitamin C, thiamine, riboflavin, niacin, calcium, and iron. Because the U.S. RDA are based on the highest values of the RDA, the former is frequently higher than the basic needs of most healthy people, though very few individuals today fall into that hypothetical category. Individuals vary by wide margins, and stress and illness, past and present, affect everyone differently. As far as I am concerned (and many other leading nutritionists), the RDA and U.S. RDA are woefully inadequate, but they are listed in sections 26–67 in the facts section for each vitamin and mineral.

126. What to Look For

When buying minerals, look for *chelated* on the label. Only 10 percent of ordinary minerals will be assimilated by the body, but when combined with amino acids in chelation, the assimilation is three to five times more efficient.

Hydrolyzed means water dispersible. *Hydrolyzed protein-chelated* means the supplement is in its most easily assimilated form.

Predigested protein is protein that has already been broken down and can go straight to the bloodstream.

Cold pressed is important to look for when buying oil or oil capsules. It means vitamins haven't been destroyed by heat and that the oil, extracted by cold-pressed methods, remains polyunsaturated.

127. Any Questions About Chapter XI?

What are emulsifiers?

Emulsifiers are used to homogenize ingredients that do not normally mix well. Lecithin and pectin, which are natural and safe, are commonly used, but unfortunately they're not used exclusively. Polysorbate 60 (which the FDA still has under investigation), locust bean (on the FDA list of additives requiring further study for mutagenic, reproductive, and teratogenic effects), and carrageenan (another being studied all too slowly by the FDA), among others, are still being used. Though these are at present generally recognized as safe (GRAS), I personally prefer and recommend products without them.

Are the dyes used in vitamin coatings natural or artificial, and how can I tell?

Regrettably, a lot of synthetic vitamins use coal-tar dyes in their coatings—and keep it a secret (in other words, there's no mention on the label). These dyes are not necessarily harmful, but they can cause allergic reactions. My advice is to play it safe and buy natural vitamins that have no artificial adulterants—and *say so!*

Are calories counted differently in foreign countries?

Most foreign countries use the metric system, and the energy value of food is measured in units called *joules,* our kilocalories, better known as calories. Four of our calories are the equivalent of seventeen joules. In other words, a joule is slightly more than four times a calorie.

XII

Your Special Vitamin Needs

128. Selecting Your Regimen

We all know that not everyone has the same metabolism, but we often forget that this also means that not everyone requires the same vitamins. In the following sections I have outlined a number of personalized regimens for a variety of specialized needs. Look them all over and see which ones best fit your own special situation. If you fall under more than one category, adjust the combined regimens so that you are not double-dosing yourself, only adding the additional vitamins.

You will notice that in many cases I advise what I call an MVP, a Mindell Vitamin Program (which can make you an MVP—a Most Valuable Player in the nutrition game). This basic vitamin trio is my foundation for general good health.

MVP MINDELL VITAMIN PROGRAM

• High-potency multiple vitamin with chelated minerals (time release preferred)
• Vitamin C, 1,000 mg. with bioflavonoids, rutin, hesperidin, and rose hips
• High-potency chelated multiple minerals

> IMPORTANT NOTE: Before starting any program, you should check "Cautions" (section 277) and with a nutritionally oriented doctor. *The regimens in this book are not prescriptive, nor are they intended as medical advice.*

129. Women

12–18 Multiple vitamin and mineral
    Vitamin C, 500 mg. with rose hips
    Vitamin E, 200 IU (dry form)
    1 of each with breakfast

19–50 MVP (see section 128)
    Vitamin E, 400 IU (dry form)
    1 of each with breakfast, and again
     with evening meal if necessary
    Also, 3 RNA-DNA 100 mg. tablets
     daily
    3 SOD tablets (see section 266) daily
     (take for only 6 days a week)
    Magnesium, 1,000 mg. and calcium,
     500 mg. daily
    Iron, 15–50 mg. daily
    1 multiple digestive enzyme when
     needed
    Stress B complex A.M. and P.M. if
     stress conditions exist

50+ MVP (see section 128)
    Vitamin E, 400 IU (dry form)
    1 of each with breakfast, and again
     at evening meal
    3 RNA-DNA 100 mg. tablets daily
    1–3 multiple digestive enzymes daily

130. Men

11–18   Multiple vitamin and mineral
Vitamin C, 500 mg. with rose hips
Vitamin E, 400 IU (dry form)
1 of each with breakfast

19–50   MVP (see section 128)
Vitamin E, 400 IU (dry form)
1 of each A.M. and P.M.
3 RNA-DNA 100 mg. tablets daily
3 SOD tablets (see section 266) daily (take
    for only 6 days a week)
Zinc, 15–50 mg. daily
Lecithin granules, 2 tbsp. or 9 capsules daily
Stress B complex A.M. and P.M. if needed

50+   MVP (see section 128)
Vitamin E, 400 IU (dry form)
1 of each twice a day
3 RNA-DNA 100 mg. tablets daily
3 SOD tablets (see section 266) daily (take
for only 6 days a week)
1–3 multiple digestive enzymes daily

131. Infants

1–4   One good-tasting chewable multiple vitamin
daily (check label to see that all the primary
vitamins are included); there should be no
artificial color, flavors, or sugar (sucrose)
added.

132. Children

4–12   Growing children need a stronger multiple vitamin containing minerals, especially calcium and iron, for normal growth. The tablet should also be high in B complex and vitamin C (50 percent of American children do not even get the RDA for vitamin C). One daily is sufficient (check label to be sure there is no artificial color, flavor, or sugar—sucrose—added).

133. Pregnant Women

The right vitamins are essential at this time:

A good high-potency multiple vitamin and mineral rich in vitamins A, B_6, B_{12}, C, and folic acid.
Multiple chelated minerals, rich in calcium (2 tablets should equal 1,000 mg. calcium and 500 mg. magnesium)
1 of each twice daily
Also, folic acid, 800 mg. 3 times a day

134. Nursing Mothers

The same supplements recommended for pregnant women plus additional vitamins A, B_6, B_{12}, and C. Your body and your baby need the best nourishment you can give them.

135. Runners

During the first fifteen to twenty minutes of running, you burn up almost only glucose. The body then comes in with fats (lipids) for energy (in utilizing lipids for energy, a compound called acetyl coenzyme A is formed). If there are only animal fats present, the compound forms slowly and energy is insufficient. If polyunsaturates are present, on the other hand, the compound forms quickly. Increase your intake of polyunsaturates— seeds, peanuts—and antioxidants, such as vitamins A, C, E, and selenium, to avoid free radical reactions.

A good supplement program would be:

Multiple vitamin with chelated minerals
Vitamin C complex, 1,000 mg.
Stress B complex with zinc
1 of each 2–3 times a day
Also, vitamin E, 400 IU A.M. and P.M. and 1 multiple chelated mineral tablet daily.
Cytochrome c and inosine, plus octacosanol 1–3 times daily

136. Joggers

The nutritional needs of joggers are the same as those for runners. Just remember: For highest energy keep polyunsaturates in mind.

137. Executives

With tension and stress an accepted part of your daily life, and energy a necessity, you need a vitamin regimen that won't let you down. Many high-level executives I know use this one:

MVP (see section 128) A.M. and P.M.
Stress B complex A.M. and P.M.
Lecithin granules, 2 tbsp. or 3 capsules with each meal
L-tryptophan, 500 mg. between meals

If you're in a hurry in the morning, you might want to try my high-energy breakfast drink:

RECIPE

2 tbsp. protein powder
1 tbsp. natural yeast
2 tbsp. lecithin granules
3 ice cubes
2 tbsp. fresh fruit, honey, or fructose

Mix in blender at high speed for one minute.

138. Students

Eating on the run, skipping breakfast, and not getting enough rest is a way of life for most students. And as if this weren't bad enough for good health, student diets usually consist mostly of starches and carbohydrates. If you're in this category, be aware that these factors, as well as your constant stress situations at school, are taking their toll. A good supplement program would be:

MVP (see section 128)
Vitamin E, 500 IU
Stress B complex with zinc
1 of each with breakfast and dinner
Choline, 100 mg. 3 times daily

Also, you might improve your work performance by increasing your intake of choline-rich foods. (See section 37.)

139. Senior Citizens

The nutritional needs of senior citizens may vary widely, depending on the individual. As a general rule, however, if you're over sixty-five, you need extra minerals, especially calcium, magnesium, and iron, as well as extra vitamins such as B complex and C. Vitamin E can help alleviate poor circulation, which is often responsible for leg cramps. And don't forget about fiber. If chewing is a problem, high-fiber foods can be ground to convenient sizes or textures and are just as effective. Also, sweets should be discouraged, as there is a high incidence of sugar diabetes among older people.

A good supplement regimen would be:

Multiple vitamin and mineral
Rose hips vitamin C, 500 mg. with bioflavonoids
Multiple chelated mineral tablet
Vitamin E, 400 IU (dry form)
1 of each with breakfast and dinner

140. Athletes

Athletes have very demanding nutritional needs. The prime nutritional requirement for performance is energy, and high-energy foods—as opposed to "quick-energy" foods—should be eaten. If you're involved in action sports, you need a diet with more complex carbohydrates and protein than someone involved in a low-energy sport. Then again, even golf can become a high-energy game when carried on intensively for a long time. Keep in mind that excess amounts of glucose, sugar, honey, or hard candy tend to draw fluid into the gastrointestinal tract. This can add to dehydration problems in endurance performance. A thirst-quenching tart drink of frozen or canned fruit juice is the best quick-energy beverage.

For supplements, I recommend:

Multiple vitamin and chelated minerals

Stress B complex
Vitamin C complex, 1,000 mg.
Vitamin E, 400–1,000 IU
Multiple chelated minerals
1 of each with breakfast, lunch, and dinner
Cytochrome c and inosine
Vitamin B_{15}, 50 mg.
Octacosanol
All 1–3 times daily

A protein supplement is also a good idea.

141. Night Workers

The Center for Research on Stress and Health at the Stanford Research Institute has found that "the rotating shift exacts a heavy physical and emotional toll from workers." When eating and sleeping patterns are disrupted, so are the body's biological rhythms, and it takes "three to four weeks for the circadian rhythms to become synchronized." If you change from day to night shifts often, your body is under much stress, your chances of illness are greater, and your risk of ulcers is high. I feel that supplements are essential:

MVP (see section 128)
1 vitamin D, 400 IU with largest meal
3 500-mg. tryptophan tablets a half hour before bedtime
(whenever that happens to be)

142. Truck Drivers

Tension, stress, and a diet that is all too often high in greasy foods are important reasons for considering the following supplements:

MVP (see section 128)
Lecithin granules, 3 tbsp. or 12 capsules daily
1 B complex, 100 mg.
3 500-mg. tryptophan tablets a half hour before bedtime
  if needed for sleep

143. Dancers

Dancers have energy requirements that rank with those of athletes, but because of weight restrictions they cannot consume the same amount of carbohydrates. Good supplements are indispensable, as most dancers will tell you. I suggest:

MVP (see section 128—be sure to take the multiple mineral twice daily)
1 balanced calcium and magnesium supplement daily

144. Construction Workers

One out of every four workers is exposed to substances considered hazardous, according to the National Institute for Occupational Safety and Health (NIOSH). Construction workers are particularly vulnerable. Depending upon the sort of construction you're doing and where you're doing it, you're exposed to a variety of harmful conditions from general pollution to inhaling lead oxide, which can happen if you're soldering scrap metal or plastics. In any event, a diet rich in antioxidants such as vitamins A, C, and E will help detoxify your body. The following supplements are recommended:

MVP (see section 128)
B complex, 100 mg. twice daily
Vitamin E, 400–1,000 IU twice daily

145. Gamblers

If you're a gambler, I don't have to tell you about your stress, sleep, and dietary needs. I'm sure you're aware that all three are higher than average. What you might not realize, though, is that you could be in need of vitamin-D supplementation because of lack of sunlight. For best performance at any table, I suggest the following supplements:

MVP (see section 128) A.M. and P.M.
Vitamin E, 400 IU twice daily
Vitamin D, 400 IU if necessary
Stress B complex with zinc

146. Salespersons

The daily grind of having to deal with the public cannot be underestimated. Whether you're selling automobiles, books, exercise machines, or food, doing it on the road or from behind a counter, the emotional and physical stress on your body is great. And because appearances are often as important as products in your line of work, you'd be wise to pack the right supplements along with your samples. You'll be happily surprised with the results.

MVP (see section 128)
Stress B complex 3 times daily (with each meal)
Vitamin E, 400 IU A.M. and P.M.

147. Actors—Radio and TV Performers

There's not an actor or actress I know who doesn't need a B-vitamin supplement. The stress and tension of performing is an occupational given. And if you're like most theatrical performers, dieting is the only form of eating you know, too often denying you necessary vitamins. A helpful supplement scenario would be:

MVP (see section 128) A.M. and P.M.
Stress B complex with zinc A.M. and P.M.
Vitamin E, 400 IU twice daily

148. Singers

Like actors, singers are also under high levels of stress, whether performing or rehearsing. If you worry about laryngitis or other throat infections, it's advisable to keep your vitamin-C levels high at all times. Time-release vitamin C is your best choice.

MVP (see section 128) A.M. and P.M.
Additional vitamin C, 1,000 mg. A.M. and P.M. when necessary

149. Doctors and Nurses

If you work with illness, you need all the protection you can get. Long hours, stress, and germs themselves all contribute to your need for vitamin and mineral supplementation.

MVP (see section 128) A.M. and P.M.
Stress B complex twice daily
Extra vitamin C to ward off infections

150. Handicapped

If you're disabled, your needs for vitamins are usually increased. More often than not, if one part of your body is not functioning properly, another part is working twice as hard—and needs nourishment. Helpful basic supplements would be:

1 B complex, 50 mg. A.M. and P.M.
1 high-potency multiple mineral twice daily

151. Golfers

As much as you enjoy it, golfing takes a lot out of you. The stress and tension of the game can use up B vitamins at a rapid clip. The right supplements might not get you down into the seventies, but they can help you stay energetic throughout the game.

MVP (see section 128) A.M. and P.M.
Stress B complex with zinc. A.M. and P.M.

152. Tennis Players

If you play tennis often, you might look good on the outside but be a nutritional mess inside. I've found that far too many tennis buffs skip meals or eat only protein— both bad habits. A demanding game like tennis requires that you serve yourself all the vitamins you need.

MVP (see section 128) A.M. and P.M.
Stress B complex A.M. and P.M.
Extra calcium to prevent muscle fatigue
Vitamin E (dry form), 400–1,000 IU daily
Wheat-germ oil

153. Racketball Players

Few sports require as intense physical stamina as racketball, so if you intend to play it on a regular basis (or even on an occasional lunch hour), you'd better be prepared to meet not only your opponent, but the nutritional challenge as well.

MVP (see section 128) A.M. and P.M.
Cytochrome c, inosine, and octacosanol twice daily
Vitamin E (dry form), 400 IU daily
Stress B complex A.M. and P.M.

154. Teachers

School days are as stressful for teachers as they are for students, if not more so. To keep your energy and spirits up, a good vitamin program is important.

MVP (see section 128) A.M. and P.M.
Stress B complex twice daily

155. Smokers

Every cigarette you smoke destroys about 25 to 100 mg. of vitamin C. Also, lung cancer risk aside, you're more prone to cardiovascular and pulmonary disorders than nonsmokers. Without going into the long list of deleterious effects cigarettes can have, I feel confident in telling smokers that they need all the nutritional help they can get, especially from antioxidants such as vitamins A, C, E, and selenium.

MVP (see section 128) A.M. and P.M.
Vitamin C, 2,000 mg. A.M. and P.M.
Vitamin E daily
Selenium 100 mcg. daily
Vitamin A, 10,000 IU daily

156. Drinkers

Alcoholism is the chief cause of vitamin deficiency among civilized people with ample food supplies. If you're a heavy drinker, the alcohol you consume usually takes the place of needed protein, or, in some cases, prevents absorption or proper storage of ingested vitamins.

MVP (see section 128) A.M. and P.M.
B complex, 100 mg. twice daily (especially needed are B_1, B_6, and folic acid)

157. Excessive TV Watchers

Just because you spend a lot of time relaxing in front of your set doesn't mean you're not in need of extra vitamins. For the eyestrain it's more than likely that you need additional vitamin A. And if you rarely get to see the light of day, you might need vitamin D, also.

MVP (see section 128) A.M. and P.M.
Vitamin A, 10,000 IU with breakfast
Vitamin D, 400 IU 5 days a week if necessary

158. Travelers on the Go

The stresses of travel, though they often go unnoticed, can be significant. If you're heading to warm or tropical places, be sure that the vitamins you take are in opaque containers and that you keep them in a cool place, not out in the sun. If you're headed for chillier environs, be sure to bring along plenty of vitamin C and take it with all your meals, not just breakfast and dinner. And if you're traveling to foreign ports, keep in mind that acidophilus (3 capsules or 2 tablespoons liquid) 3 times a day is a good diarrhea preventive.

MVP (see section 128) A.M. and P.M.
Vitamin E (dry form), 400 IU 1–2 times daily
Stress B complex, 50 mg. 2–3 times daily

159. Any Questions About Chapter XII?

Are foreign vitamins different?

Vitamins the world over are the same, only dosages vary. The metric system is used internationally for measurement, and nutrients are measured by weight. (See section 124 for a better understanding of what equals what.)

My obstetrician doesn't say too much to me, except "Take your vitamins." Since you're a pharmacist as well as a nutritionist, could you tell me what drugs or medicines could be dangerous to me and my baby?

I'd feel safest in saying all of them—unless specifically prescribed by your doctor. No drug—whether it's OTC (over the counter) or prescription, alcohol, nicotine, or caffeine—should be considered safe during pregnancy. Most drugs can cross the placenta and thus affect fetus as well as mother. Considering that the major stages in an embryo's development occur during life's first few weeks, if you're even *thinking* about being a mother, check with your doctor before taking any medication.

Are older people subject to any specific nutrient deficiencies?

As a general rule they are. Aside from the fact that they consume more drugs than any other age group, they usually suffer from subclinical nutritional deficiencies because of their life-style and marginal intakes of key nutrients caused by malabsorption, poor teeth, loneliness, and other social problems. Their most common nutrient deficiencies are folic acid, calcium, vitamin B_{12}, vitamin D, and vitamin C.

XIII

The Right Vitamin at the Right Time

160. Special Situation Supplements

Your body's vitamin needs are not always the same, and special situations require special food regimens and supplements. What follows is a list of such situations, most of them temporary, with supplement suggestions. For foods that offer specific vitamins and minerals, see sections 26 through 67. Once again, this information is not prescriptive. (See section 128 for MVP.)

161. Acne

This scourge of teenage years has been treated in a variety of ways, from X rays to tetracycline, with only varying degrees of success. I encourage more natural treatment of the condition and have been delighted by the results.

Multiple vitamin with minerals, but low in iodine (iodine can worsen acne conditions), 1 daily
Vitamin E (dry form), 400 IU 1–2 times daily
Vitamin A, 25,000 IU (water soluble) 1–2 times daily, 5 days a week

Zinc, 50 mg. chelated, 1 tablet 3 times daily with meals
Acidophilus liquid, 1–2 tbsp. or 3–6 capsules 3 times
  daily
(Eliminate all processed foods. They are usually high in
  salt that has been iodized.)

162. Athlete's Foot

Vitamin-C powder or crystals applied directly to the
affected areas seems to help this fungus infection. Keep
your feet dry and out of shoes as much as possible until
the infection clears.

163. Bad Breath

Along with proper brushing and flossing, you might try:

MVP (see section 128)
1 chlorophyll tablet or capsule 1–3 times daily
3 acidophilus capsules or 1–2 tbsp. flavored acidophilus
  3 times daily
Zinc, 50 mg. 1–3 times daily

164. Baldness or Falling Hair

There are no guarantees, but many people report a
definite diminution of hair loss with this regimen:

Stress B complex twice daily
Choline and inositol, 1,000 mg. of each daily
Daily jojoba oil scalp massage and shampoo
A multiple-mineral formula with 1,000 mg. calcium and
  500 mg. magnesium, 1 daily
Cysteine, 1,000 mg. daily
Vitamin C, 1,000 mg. 3 times daily

165. Bee Stings

The best thing to do about bee stings is try to avoid them. Vitamin B_1 (thiamine) has been shown to be a fairly good insect repellent. Taken three times daily, 100 mg. B_1 creates a smell at the level of your skin that insects do not like. If you're too late with the B_1 and do get stung, 1,000 mg. vitamin C could help ease allergic reactions.

166. Bleeding Gums

The most effective vitamin therapy for bleeding gums is 1,000 mg. vitamin C complex, with bioflavonoids, rutin, and hesperidin, taken three times a day.

167. Broken Bones

If you've ever broken a bone, you know how frustrating it is waiting for it to mend. That feeling can be alleviated, and bone healing accelerated, by increasing your calcium and vitamin-D intakes. Daily doses of 1,000–1,500 mg. calcium and 400–500 IU vitamin D are good.

168. Bruises

Vitamin C complex, 1,000 mg. with bioflavonoids, rutin, and hesperidin, taken three times daily will help prevent capillary fragility, those black-and-blue marks that occur when the tiny blood vessels beneath the skin rupture.

169. Burns

The most important thing to do with a burn is to put cold water on it immediately. To effectively stimulate wound healing, 50 mg. zinc daily has been found useful and is worth trying. Vitamin C complex, 1,000 mg. with bioflavonoids, taken in the morning and evening is recommended to prevent infections. Vitamin E, 1,000 IU, used orally and topically can help prevent scarring.

170. Cold Feet

If you're embarrassed by wearing socks to bed all the time, you could try a good multimineral supplement with iodine twice a day, along with kelp tablets. The cold feet could be caused by the fact that your thyroid glands are not producing enough thyroxine. Niacin and vitamin E can also help circulation.

171. Cold Sores and Herpex Simplex

Few things are more annoying than cold sores. The best supplement remedy I've discovered is:

Vitamin C complex, 1,000 mg. with bioflavonaoids A.M. and P.M.
Lactobacillus acidophilus, 3 capsules 3 times a day
Vitamin-E oil, 28,000 IU applied directly to affected area
Lysine, 3 g. (3,000 mg.) 3 times daily (in divided doses) between meals (with water or juice—no protein)
As a preventive: Lysine, 500 mg. daily (with water or juice—no protein)
Vitamin C, 1,000 mg. A.M. and P.M.

172. Constipation

Everyone is bothered by constipation at some time or other. Usually this is caused by a lack of bulk in the diet or because of certain medications, such as codeine. Harsh laxatives can rob the body of nutrients, as well as cause rebound constipation and laxative dependency, so natural remedies should be your first choice.

2 tbsp. unprocessed bran flakes 1–3 times daily or 3–9 bran tablets 3 times daily

1 tbsp. acidophilus liquid 3 times daily

A vegetable laxative and sugar-free stool softener for a short time if necessary

8–10 glasses of water daily (and a little exercise wouldn't hurt)

173. Cuts

Vitamin C complex, 1,000 mg. with bioflavonoids twice daily, along with 50 mg. zinc and 1,000 IU vitamin E.

174. Dry Skin

Vitamin-E oil seems to work wonders when applied to dry skin, as do oils rich in vitamins A and D. As a dietary supplement, if you're not eating enough sweet potatoes, carrots, liver, and tomatoes, try 25,000 IU vitamin A daily for two weeks, then cut dosage back to 10,000 IU. If you've cut all fats from your diet, put some back in the form of polyunsaturated oil (2 table-spoons on your daily salad is ample). Or try 3 to 6 lecithin capsules three times daily, along with the MVP. Another alternative is 1 tbsp. cod liver oil (flavored) taken with milk or juice one hour before breakfast.

175. Hangovers

To prevent them, take 1 B complex, 100 mg., before going out, 1 again while you're drinking, and another right before going to bed (alcohol destroys B complex). Cysteine, 500 mg., with vitamin C, 1,500 mg., can help, too.

176. Hay Fever

Stress can cause hay fever attacks to worsen. If you're one of the many who suffer, you might find relief with 1 stress B complex twice daily, 1,000 mg. pantothenic acid three times daily, and the same dose of vitamin C, which has evidenced effective antihistamine properties.

177. Headaches

A surprisingly effective vitamin-mineral regimen for headaches is:

100 mg. niacin 3 times daily
100 mg. stress B complex (time release) twice daily
Calcium and magnesium (twice as much calcium as magnesium is the proper ratio), which are nature's tranquilizers

178. Heartburn

Over-the-counter antacids, such as Gelusil, Winger, Kolantyl, Maalox, Di-Gel, and Rolaids, contain aluminum, which disturbs calcium and phosphorus metabolism. You'll probably be better off taking 5 bonemeal tablets daily (with food), multiple digestive enzymes one to three times daily, and chewable papaya and drinking fluids before or after meals, *not* during.

179. Hemorrhoids

Just about half the people over fifty are afflicted by hemorrhoids. Improper diet, lack of exercise, and straining at stool are all contributing factors (and coffee, chocolate, cola, and cocoa are accessories to the discomfort by promoting anal itching). If you're bothered by hemorrhoids, 1 tablespoon of unprocessed bran three times a day is helpful, along with 1,000 mg. vitamin C complex twice a day for healing membranes, and 3 acidophilus capsules three times a day (or 1 to 2 tablespoons of acidophilus liquid one to three times a day). Vitamin-E oil, 28,000 IU per ounce, can be applied to the affected area with a cotton swab.

180. Insomnia

Barbiturates, such as phenobarbital, Seconal, Nembutal, and Butisol, are strong sedatives and hypnotics that are too often prescribed for insomnia. Aside from being habit-forming and dangerous if mixed with other drugs, these barbiturates can also cause low calcium levels.

Tryptophan, on the other hand, is a natural amino acid that is essential to our bodies and can help induce sleep.

An effective insomnia program:

3 tryptophan tablets (500–667 mg.) ½ hour before bedtime with water or juice
1 chelated calcium and magnesium tablet 3 times daily and 3 tablets ½ hour before bedtime
Vitamin B_6 and niacinamide, 100 mg. each, work together to produce the brain chemical serotonin, which is essential for restful REM sleep.

Milk, as you know, is a fine natural source of calcium, and turkey is a good source of tryptophan. An open-face turkey sandwich and a glass of warm milk before bedtime could be the sleep remedy of your life.

(If you tend to wake in the middle of the night, take 500–667 mg. of tryptophan 1½ hours before bedtime.)

181. Itching

As an antihistamine, 2 1,000-mg. vitamin-C tablets (time release) in the morning and evening, with food, might be helpful. I would also recommend a stress B complex with breakfast and dinner, 1,000 mg. pantothenic acid one to three times daily, and vitamin-E cream (25,000 IU per ounce) applied to the afflicted area three times daily.

182. Jet Lag

So your plane from London lands at 9 A.M. and you're supposed to be at a meeting at 10 A.M. No problem, except for the fact that as far as your body is concerned, it's still only 4 A.M. and you should be asleep. Your best bet is to help your system catch up with your schedule by giving it the vitamins it needs.

Stress B complex (time release A.M. and P.M. Start while still on the plane.)
MVP with food, twice during flights of five or more hours
Vitamin E, 400 IU twice daily

If you're feeling run-down, as well as tired, be sure to take additional vitamin C.

183. Leg Pains

Increase your calcium. Try 1 chelated calcium and magnesium tablet with breakfast and dinner, along with a chelated multiple mineral. Vitamin E has been reported quite helpful in cases of charley horse. The most common doses for it are 400 to 1,000 IU (dry form) one to three times daily.

184. Menopause

Because of the risks that have recently been brought to light about estrogens, many women have been seeking other ways to relieve the discomforts of menopause. A good number of menopausal women have found that 400 IU vitamin E (mixed tocopherols) one to three times a day does indeed alleviate hot flashes. If you're at that time of life, MVP and a 600-mg. stress B complex twice a day also seem to help. Ginseng, 500 mg., and damiana taken 1–3 times daily before meals have been successful, too.

185. Menstruation

Between the cramps and the bloating, menstruation is for most women a monthly annoyance. But this annoyance can dwindle to a mere distraction once the discomfort is alleviated.

Vitamin B$_6$, 150 mg. 3 times daily (most effective as a natural diuretic)
B complex, 100 mg. (time release) A.M. and P.M.
MVP
Evening primrose oil, 500 mg. 3 times daily

186. Motion Sickness

This is one condition where remedies are most effective if taken beforehand. Vitamins B_1 and B_6 are the nutrients of choice (in fact, many prenatal antinausea preparations contain vitamin B_6). Taking 100 mg. B complex the night before you leave and the morning of your trip has been found to be effective by many queasy travelers. Ginger root capsules taken three times daily work, also!

187. Muscle Soreness

For that ache-all-over feeling after a workout or just general muscle soreness, I've seen many people find relief with vitamin E, 400 to 1,000 IU taken one to three times daily. A chelated multiple mineral in the morning and at night also has helped.

188. The Pill

If you take oral contraceptives, not only are you more vulnerable than other women to blood clots, strokes, and heart attacks, but you're also more likely to be deficient in zinc, folic acid, vitamins C, B_6, and B_{12} (which accounts for much nervousness and depression among pill takers).

Supplements are important:

MVP
Zinc, 50 mg. chelated, 1–3 tablets daily
Folic acid, 800 mcg. 1–3 times daily
B_{12}, 2,000 mcg. (time release or sublingual), A.M.
B_6, 150 mg. 1–3 times daily

189. Poison Ivy

Vitamin-E oil or aloe vera gel applied externally can help healing. Two 1,000-mg. vitamin C complex (time release) taken A.M. and P.M. along with vitamin E, 400 to 1,000 IU, should alleviate the itching.

190. Polyps

These small annoying growths could be a possible cancer risk and should definitely be checked by a doctor, and in most instances surgical removal is necessary. But as far as supplements go, Dr. Jerome J. DeCosse, professor and chairman of surgery at the Medical College of Wisconsin, used 3,000 mg. vitamin C (time release) daily on patients with polyps and had noteworthy success with the treatment.

191. Postoperative Healing

After surgery, your body needs all the nutritional support it can get.

Vitamin E, 400 IU (dry form) 3 times daily
2 vitamin C complex, 1,000 mg. with bioflavonoids, hesperidin, and rutin A.M. and P.M.
High-potency multiple vitamin with chelated minerals A.M. and P.M.
High-potency multiple chelated mineral tablet A.M. and P.M.
Vitamin A, 10,000–25,000 IU 3 times daily for 5 days (stop for 2 days to prevent buildup)
Chelated zinc, 15–50 mg. daily

192. Prickly Heat

Much like itching, prickly heat seems to respond to the antihistamine properties of vitamin C. (See section 181 for regimen.)

193. Prostate Problems

Chronic prostatitis, has been found to respond to treatment with zinc. (The prostate gland normally contains about ten times more zinc than any other organ in the body.) In many cases, symptoms have completely disappeared with adherence to the following regimen:

MVP
Chelated zinc, 50 mg. 3 times daily
Vitamin F or lecithin capsules (1,200 mg.), 3 caps 3
    times daily

194. Psoriasis

Though many jokes have been made about this disease, it is no laughing matter to the millions who suffer from it. No one treatment has been found to be totally effective, but the following has met with much success:

MVP
Vitamin A (water soluble), 10,000 IU 3 times daily for
    5 days a week
B complex, 100 mg. (time release) A.M. and P.M.
Rose hips vitamin C, 1,000 mg. A.M. and P.M. (this is
    in addition to the vitamin C called for in the MVP)
Vitamin E (dry form), 400 IU 3 times daily
3 vitamin-F or lecithin capsules 3 times daily
Increase protein (preferably animal source)

195. Stopping Smoking

It's no mean feat to stop smoking, and your body knows it. Those withdrawal symptoms are real. For the irritability that occurs, 1 tryptophan (550–667 mg.) tablet three times a day between meals seems to help. Also take 1 B complex, 100 mg. (time release), with the evening meal, and 100 mg. cysteine with 300 mg. vitamin C daily. And don't forget your MVP.

196. Sunburn

A good sunscreening preparation should always be used before exposing yourself to the sun's ultraviolet rays for any length of time. What most people don't realize is that the sun actually burns the skin, and bad burns can break the skin and leave it vulnerable to infection.

If it's too late for preventives, try this:

Aloe vera gel applied 3–4 times daily
A PABA cream or vitamin-E cream (20,000 IU) also
    applied 3–4 times daily
MVP
Additional vitamin C, 1,000 mg. A.M. and P.M. until
    burn heals

197. Teeth Grinding

People are usually unaware of grinding their teeth. It occurs more often in children than adults and most often during sleep. MVP; B complex, 100 mg. A.M. and P.M.; and a few bonemeal tablets nightly before sleep can help.

198. Varicose Veins

Age, lack of exercise, and chronic constipation are contributing factors to varicose veins. Watching your diet and exercising regularly can do a lot toward preventing them. MVP with an extra 1,000 mg. vitamin C complex twice daily has been found to help, along with 400 to 800 IU vitamin E.

199. Vasectomy

Men with vasectomies are more susceptible to infections and would be wise to take an additional 1,000 mg. vitamin C complex daily, along with regular MVP diet supplementation. Extra zinc, 15–50 mg. every day, is also a good idea.

200. Warts

They don't come from handling frogs, but they do seem to effectively disappear when treated with vitamin-E oil. The most successful regimen appears to be 28,000 IU vitamin E applied externally one to two times daily and 400 IU vitamin E (dry form) taken internally three times a day. Vitamin C complex, 1,000–2,000 mg. daily, can help build up the body's immunity and possibly prevent warts from occurring at all.

201. Any Questions About Chapter XIII?

You talk about digestive enzymes being helpful for heartburn. What are they and what do they do?

Enzymes, which can be purchased as supplements, can help your own digestive system assimilate the foods you eat. *Bromelain,* for instance, is a digestive enzyme from pineapple. *Cellulose* is an aid to digesting vegetable matter and breaking down food fiber. *Hydrochloric acid (HCl)* works in the stomach on tough foods, such as fibrous meats, vegetables, and poultry (betaine HCl is the best form available). *Lipase* assists in fat digestion and *mylase* dissolves thousands of times its own weight in starches so you can more easily assimilate them. *Papain* is a protein-digesting enzyme (from papaya), and *prolase* is a concentrated protein-digesting enzyme derived from papain (see section 178).

Is there a specific reason for your recommending ginseng in the treatment of menopause?

Definitely. Since estrogen replacement began in the 1960s, it has been linked to a 35 percent increase in uterine cancer. Ginseng contains estriol, an anticarcinogenic (cancer-fighting) variant of estrogen.

XIV

Getting Well and Staying That Way

202. Why You Need Supplements During Illness

During illness the body is under stress. Cells are destroyed, exhausted adrenal glands deprived of nutrients are unable to function properly, and the body's stress-fighting team of vitamin C, vitamin B_6, folic acid, and pantothenic acid is severely depleted (zinc and vitamin E are also needed in greater amounts).

Because we require these vitamins to effectively utilize other nutrients and to keep our metabolism functioning all the time, our need for them is obviously increased when we're ill. And since we know that fever and stress rob our body of its most essential nutrients, the importance of supplements is self-evident.

Again, *the following regimens are not intended as medical advice, only as a guide in working with your doctor.*

203. Allergies

Allergies come in all shapes and sizes, with all sorts of symptoms, and you can contract them for just about anything. Nonetheless they take their nutritional toll, and supplements can help.

MVP (see section 128) A.M. and P.M.
Vitamin B complex, 100 mg. 3 times daily
Pantothenic acid, 1,000 mg. A.M. and P.M.

If you have an allergy, it would be a good idea to take a hard look at your present diet. Many allergies are caused by MSG, food coloring, additives, and preservatives.

204. Arthritis

Thousands of people suffer from this painful chronic condition. Because it puts so much stress on the body, vitamin-mineral supplementation is really essential.

MVP (see section 128)
Extra vitamin C, 1,000 mg. 1–3 times a day (if you're taking lots of aspirin, you're losing vitamin C)
B complex, 100 mg. 1–3 times a day
B_{12}, up to 2,000 mcg. daily
Niacin up to 1 g. daily
1–3 yucca tabs 3 times daily
Pantothenic acid, 100 mg. 3 times daily
Cod liver oil, 1–2 tbsp. 3 times daily (if capsules, 3 caps 3 times daily); take for 5 days and stop for 2

205. Asthma

Asthma is a chronic allergic condition that affects the bronchial tubes, and warrants medical attention. When an attack occurs, the muscle tissue of the tubes constricts spasmodically, squeezing the air passages and causing labored breathing and a feeling of suffocation. Allergies, heredity, and emotional stress have all been implicated as contributing factors to asthmatic conditions, but many nutrients have been found to provide remarkable natural relief, though they should not be considered as substitutes for professional medical care.

MVP (see section 128) A.M. and P.M.

Extra vitamin C, 1,000 mg. 1–3 times daily
(CAUTION: Vitamin C that's buffered with calcium ascorbate can interefere with the action of tetracylines. A sodium ascorbate form of vitamin C can be used with tetracyclines, but not if you are on a sodium-restricted diet or are taking steroids.)

Evening primrose oil, 2 500-mg. tablets 3 times daily for 3 to 4 months; then 1 tablet 3 times daily
(If you are taking steroids, you won't benefit from EPO, because steroids interfere with EPO's action.)

Glandulars (adrenal gland concentrates) 1–3 times daily, but not at night, because they might cause insomnia
(CAUTION: Glandulars should not be taken by anyone who is allergic to beef or pork.)

Vitamin A (water soluble), 10,000–25,000 IU daily
Vitamin B_2 (riboflavin), 100 mg. 3–4 times daily
Vitamin B_5 (pantothenic acid), 1,000–2,000 mg. daily
Vitamin B_6 (pyridoxine), 100–200 mg. 1–4 times daily
Vitamin E (dry form), 400–1,200 IU daily

206. Blood Pressure—High and Low

HIGH

Over sixty million Americans have high blood pressure, which has been intimately linked to heart attacks and strokes. The importance of keeping your blood pressure down cannot be overestimated, and there are a number of natural ways that can help.

• Talk slower (fast talkers often don't breathe properly and this can result in elevated blood pressure).
• Reduce, if you are overweight (controlled, sensible dieting can significantly lower blood pressure in overweight individuals).
• Decrease sodium and increase potassium in your diet (see section 257 on hidden salt in foods).
• Decrease your sugar intake (see section 255).
• Eliminate caffeine (see sections 229 and 230).
• Eat more onions and garlic.
• Stop smoking.
• Avoid stress or anxiety-provoking situations (jangling everyday noises, even loud televisions, can cause stress and elevate blood pressure).
• Get regular exercise (such as brisk walking) and adequate rest.

Regimen

Lecithin granules, 3 tbsp. daily, or 3 caps 3 times daily
Potassium may be necessary if you are taking an antihypertensive, but check with your doctor to be sure it's not contraindicated for your particular medication
MVP (see section 128)
Calcium, 1,000–1,500 mg. daily

Vitamin E, 100 IU daily and work up to higher strengths (check with your doctor)
Garlic perles (deodorized) 1–3 daily

LOW

Low blood pressure, unless extreme, is a far better condition to have than its alternative. Nonetheless, hypotensives often suffer from dizziness and occasional fainting spells and blackouts.

Regimen
1–3 kelp tablets daily
 (NOTE: If you're taking thyroid medication, check with your doctor, as kelp might decrease the need for the amount you're currently taking.)
MVP (see section 128)

207. Bronchitis

This inflammation of the bronchial tube lining is quite common and extremely enervating. The stress it puts on the body is high, and even antibiotics are the bad guys as far as nutrients are concerned. (See section 239.)

Vitamin A, 25,000 IU 1–3 times daily (take for 5 days, then stop for 2)
Rose hips vitamin C, 1,000 mg. A.M. and P.M.
MVP (see section 128)
Vitamin E (dry form), 400 IU 1–3 times daily
Water, 6–8 glasses daily
3 acidophilus caps or 1–2 tbsp. liquid 3 times daily

208. Chicken Pox

This childhood staple is caused by a virus closely related to that of shingles. The fever and itching deplete a good amount of nutrients. Many mothers have found their children up and about faster by adding the following supplements to their diets.

Rose hips vitamin C, 500 mg. 3 times daily
Vitamin E, 100–200 IU 1–3 times daily
Vitamin A, 10,000 IU daily (check pediatrician for proper dosage according to age and weight); take for 5 days and stop for 2
Multivitamin and multimineral A.M. and P.M.

209. Colds

No one pays too much attention to a cold, except the body—it pays plenty.

MVP (see section 128)
Rose hips vitamin C, 1,000 mg. 3 times daily
Vitamin A, 25,000 IU 1–3 times daily (take for 5 days and stop for 2)
Vitamin E (dry form), 200–400 IU daily
Water, 6–8 glasses daily
3 acidophilus caps or 1–2 tbsp. liquid 3 times daily
1 zinc lozenge, 15 mg. 3 times daily.

210. Colitis

As a rule this illness is more common in women than men and often is triggered by emotional upset. Alternating diarrhea and constipation, as well as abdominal pain, are its distressing hallmarks. Diet is of prime importance and vitamins are recommended.

MVP (see section 128)
Potassium, 99 mg. (elemental) 1–3 times daily
Raw cabbage juice (vitamin U), 1 glass 3 times daily
Water, 6–8 glasses daily
Aloe vera gel (for internal use), 1 tbsp. 3 times daily or
    1–3 capsules 3 times daily
3–6 acidophilus caps or 2 tbsp. liquid 3 times daily
1 tbsp. bran flakes or 3–6 bran tablets 3 times daily

211. Diabetes

What happens in diabetes, primarily, is that the pancreas
fails to produce adequate insulin and the blood sugar
rises uncontrollably. In mild cases diet alone can control
the condition. (Beware of hidden sugars. See section
255.) In severe cases, replacement insulin is necessary.
In all cases, the care of a physician is essential.

   Supplements that have aided diabetics are:

MVP (see section 128)
Glucose tolerance factor (GTF) chromium, 200 mcg. 1–3
    times daily
Potassium, 99 mg. 3 times daily
Chelated zinc, 50 mg. 1–3 times daily
Water, 6–8 glasses daily
    (CAUTION: The combination of vitamin B_1, vitamin
    C, and cysteine has the potential to reduce insulin
    effectiveness for diabetics, and should only be taken
    under medical supervision.)

212. Eye Problems

From simple inflammations to refraction difficulties to
serious diseases, eye problems should never be ignored,
nor should visits to the ophthalmologist be postponed.

There are, however, generally beneficial supplements you can take.

Vitamin A, 10,000 IU 1–3 times daily (take for 5 days, then stop for 2)
B complex, 100 mg. (time release) A.M. and P.M.
Rose hips vitamin C complex, 500 mg. A.M. and P.M.
Vitamin E (dry form), 400 IU A.M. and P.M.

213. Heart Conditions

With any heart condition, you should be under a doctor's care. Though the following supplements have been found to be quite safe and helpful, you should check with your physician to make sure they are not contra-indicated in your particular case. (Vitamin E can increase the imbalance between the two sides of the heart for some people with rheumatic hearts.)

Vitamin B, 100 mg. (time release) A.M. and P.M.
Extra niacin, 100 mg. 1–3 times daily
Vitamin E (dry form), 400 IU daily
MVP (see section 128)
3 lecithin capsules or 3 tbsp. granules 3 times daily

HEART ATTACK PREVENTION TACTICS
• Decrease sugar and salt consumption.
• Stop smoking.
• Exercise regularly.
• Watch your weight.
• Practice relaxation techniques such as meditation and biofeedback to reduce stress.

• Decrease intake of saturated fats, hydrogenated oils, and cholesterol.

• Eat more garlic, fresh fruit, and fish.

• Increase your soy protein intake (use in place of animal protein whenever possible).

• Get enough calcium and magnesium in your diet (supplements of 1,000 mg. calcium and 500 mg. magnesium daily are recommended).

• Be sure you're getting enough vitamins C, B_6, and E.

• Supplement lecithin in your diet.

• Laughter is great medicine (not only does it release pent-up emotions and stress . . . it's fun and feels good, too).

214. Hypoglycemia

Though an estimated 20 to 40 million Americans have it, this disease is one of the most often undiagnosed. It is a condition of low blood sugar and, like diabetes, presents a situation where the body is unable to metabolize carbohydrates normally. Since a hypoglycemic's system overreacts to sugar, producing too much insulin, the key to raising blood sugar levels is not by eating rapidly metabolized carbohydrates, but by eating more protein.

Recommended supplements:

Vitamin A and D capsules (10,000 and 400 IU) 1–3 times daily for 5 days, then stop for 2

Vitamin C, 500 mg. with or after each meal

Vitamin E, 100–200 IU 3 times daily

B complex, 50 mg. 3 times daily

Vitamin F, 1 capsule 3 times daily

Multiple mineral tab A.M. and P.M. (niacin as needed and tolerated; see section 44)
Pantothenic acid, 500 mg. twice daily
2 lecithin capsules (19 grains = 1,200 mg.) 3 times daily
Digestive enzymes if necessary
1 kelp tablet 3 times daily
3 acidophilus capsules or 1–2 tbsp. liquid 3 times daily
GTF chromium, 50 mg. 3 times daily

215. Impetigo

Caused by germs similar to those that cause boils—staphylococcus or streptococcus—it occurs more in children than adults, but no one is immune. It often results from scratching and infecting insect bites, allowing the germs to get into broken skin.

Vitamin A and D capsules (10,000 and 400 IU) 1–3 times daily (reduce dose for children) for 5 days, then stop for 2
Vitamin E (dry form), 100–400 IU once a day
Rose hips vitamin C, 500 mg. A.M. and P.M.

216. Measles

You can get measles at any age, though it's more common among children. It is the most contagious of the communicable diseases. There is now a preventive vaccine for it, but the virus still manages to get a large number of the unprotected each year. The disease and rash can be mild or severe with a heavy cough. Your body needs vitamins to help fight and recover from it.

Vitamin A, 10,000 IU (reduce dose for children) 1–3 times daily for 5 days, then stop for 2

Rose hips vitamin C, 500–1,000 mg. A.M. and P.M.
Vitamin E (dry form), 200–400 IU A.M. and P.M.

217. Mononucleosis

Commonly contracted by adolescents and young adults, mono (glandular fever) or "the kissing disease," as it is often called, can happen to anyone and can deplete the body of massive amounts of nutrients.

Diet is important and supplements are generally considered essential during the long convalescence.

MVP (see section 128) A.M. and P.M.
Extra vitamin C, 1,000 mg. A.M. and P.M. for 3 months
Potassium, 99 mg. 3 times daily
B complex, 100 mg. (time release) A.M. and P.M.

218. Mumps

A vaccine for mumps exists, but the disease is still quite common and just as nutritionally debilitating. The virus can spread through the patient's entire system, involving not only the salivary glands but the testicles or ovaries, the pancreas, the nervous system, and sometimes even the heart.

Vitamin A, 10,000 IU (reduce does for children) 1–3
    times daily for 5 days, then stop for 2
Rose hips vitamin C, 500–1,000 mg. twice daily
Vitamin E, 200–400 IU (dry form) daily

219. PMS (Premenstrual Syndrome)

For two to ten days before the onset of menstruation, millions of women are affected by a wide range of physical discomforts and mood disorders—from bloating, depression, and insomnia to severe pains, uncontrolled rages, crying spells, and even suicidal depression. This is know as PMS, premenstrual syndrome.

FOODS AND BEVERAGES TO AVOID

• Salt and salty foods (see section 258).

• Licorice (it stimulates the production of aldosterone, which causes further retention of sodium and water).

• Cold foods and beverages (these adversely affect abdominal circulation and worsen cramping).

• Caffeine in all forms (see section 230). Caffeine increases the craving for sugar, wastes B vitamins, washes out potassium and zinc, and increases hydrochloric acid (HC1) sections, which can cause abdominal irritation.

• Astringent dark teas (tannin binds important minerals and prevents absorption in the digestive tract).

• Alcohol (adversely affects blood sugar, depletes magnesium levels, and can interfere with proper liver function, which can aggravate PMS).

• Spinach, beet greens, and other oxalate-containing vegetables (oxalates make minerals nonassimilable, difficult to be properly absorbed).

FOODS AND BEVERAGES TO INCREASE

• Strawberries, watermelon (eat seeds), artichokes, asparagus, parsley and watercress (these are natural diuretics).

• Raw sunflower seeds, dates, figs, peaches, bananas, potatoes, peanuts, and tomatoes (rich in potassium).

• Try Dong Quai; it's an herb known as the female

ginseng and can improve circulation, regulate liver function, and help remove excess water from the system.

Suggested supplements

Vitamin B₆, 50–300 mg. daily (work up from 50 mg. gradually)

MVP (see section 128)

Magnesium, 500 mg., and calcium, 250 mg., daily (Yes, with PMS it is twice as much magnesium as calcium, because a magnesium deficiency causes many of the PMS symptoms.)

Vitamin E (dry form), 100–400 IU daily

Pantothenic acid (vitamin B), 1,000 mg. (1 g.) daily

Evening primrose oil, 500 mg. 1–3 times daily

And exercise! Aside from the fact that this will improve abdominal circulation, perspiration helps remove excess fluids. Brisk walking for thirty minutes twice daily and/or swimming are highly recommended.

220. Shingles

Shingles (herpes zoster) is caused by a virus much like the one that causes chicken pox. But where chicken pox causes a general skin eruption, shingles usually erupts along a nerve path. Differences aside, the nutritional deficit caused by both diseases is high.

Vitamin A, 10,000–25,000 IU daily for 5 days, then stop for 2

Vitamin B complex, 100 mg. (time release) A.M. and P.M.

Rose hips vitamin C with bioflavonoids, 1,000–2,000 mg. A.M. and P.M.

Vitamin D, 1,000 IU daily for 5 days, then stop for 2

221. Tonsillitis

An inflammation of the tonsils that can afflict any age group, though it is more common in children. Good nutrition and supplements have been effective in preventing it as well as recovering from it.

MVP (see section 128) A.M. and P.M. with food
Vitamin A, 10,000–25,000 IU (reduce dose for children) 1–3 times daily for 5 days, then stop for 2
Extra vitamin C complex, 1,000 mg. A.M. and P.M.
Vitamin E (dry form), 200–400 IU daily
3 acidophilus caps or 1–2 tbsp. 3 times daily
Water, 6–8 glasses daily

222. Ulcers

There are two types of peptic ulcers, one in the stomach and the other in the duodenum, usually associated with excessive acidity in the stomach juices (see section 9). For both of these conditions, supplements have been found helpful.

Vitamin A, 25,000 IU 1–3 times daily for 5 days, then stop for 2
Vitamin B complex, 100 mg. (time release) A.M. and P.M.
Rose hips vitamin C with bioflavonoids, 1,000 mg. (time release) A.M. and P.M.
High-potency multiple mineral A.M. and P.M.
Aloe vera gel, 1–3 capsules or 1–3 tbsp. liquid daily

223. Veneral Disease

Syphilis and gonorrhea are still the main types of venereal disease, and though sulfa drugs, penicillin, tetracycline, erythromycin, and newer antibiotics are the most effective treatments for them, these remedies cause almost as much need for supplements as the diseases themselves.

MVP (see section 128)
3 acidophilus caps or 1–2 tbsp. liquid 3 times daily
Extra vitamin C, 1,000 mg. A.M. and P.M.
Vitamin K, 100 mcg. daily if on extended antibiotic program

Genital herpes has become American's number-one veneral disease of the eighties. Like herpes simplex type I, which causes cold sores (see section 171), type II herpes, which causes genital infection, also seems to respond well to lysine-rich foods. As a preventative, it wouldn't be a bad idea to increase your intake of cottage cheese, flounder, tuna fish, peanuts, raw chick peas (garbanzos), and soybeans. *Acyclovir* (Zovirax) is a drug that—at this writing—seems to be effective in blocking herpes replication, but the final results are not yet in. Meanwhile, I'd suggest a preventative supplement of lysine, 500 mg. daily (with water or juice—no protein) and vitamin C, 1,000 mg. A.M. and P.M. If you already have the virus: lysine, 3 g. (3,000 mg.) 3 times daily—in divided doses—between meals.

CAUTION: If you have symptoms of herpes simplex I or II, avoid supplementation of arginine and arginine-rich foods (see section 80).

224. Any Questions About Chapter XIV?

When you talk about blood pressure, what's normal and what's "high"?

You are considered within normal range if your higher (systolic) pressure is between 100 and 140, and your lower (diastolic) pressure is in the range of 60 to 90. For a healthy young adult, a reading of 120/80 is considered normal.

XV

It's Not All in Your Mind

225. How Vitamins and Minerals Affect Your Moods

The first scientifically documented discovery to relate mental illness to diet occurred when it was found that pellagra (with its depression, diarrhea, and dementia) could be cured with niacin. After that, it was shown that supplementation with the whole B complex produced greater benefits than niacin alone.

Evidence of biochemical causes for mental disturbances continues to mount. Experiments have shown that symptoms of mental illness can be switched off and on by altering vitamin levels in the body.

> Even normal, happy people can become depressed when made deficient in niacin or folic acid.

Dr. R. Shulman, reporting in the *British Journal of Psychiatry,* found that forty-eight out of fifty-nine psychiatric patients had folic-acid deficiencies. Other research has shown that the majority of the mentally and emotionally ill are deficient in one or more of the

B-complex vitamins or vitamin C. Even normal, happy people have been found to become depressed and experience other symptoms of emotional disturbance when made niacin or folic-acid deficient.

At California's Stanford University, Dr. Linus Pauling conducted a series of tests to determine individual vitamin needs. As part of the series, he administered massive doses of vitamin C (as much as 40 g.) to schizophrenics and discovered that little or none of it was discarded in the urine. Since the body expels what it doesn't need of the water-soluble vitamins, the test clearly indicated that the mentally ill needed more vitamin C—more than one thousand times the RDA—than the rest of us.

226. Vitamins and Minerals for Depression and Anxiety

The following vitamins and minerals have in many cases been found to be effective in the treatment of depression and anxiety.

Vitamin B_1 (thiamine)—large amounts appear to energize depressed people and tranquilize anxious ones

Vitamin B_6 (pyridoxine)—important for the function of the adrenal cortex

Pantothenic acid—has a tension-relieving effect

Vitamin C (ascorbic acid)—essential for combating stress

Vitamin E (alpha-tocopherol)—aids brain cells in getting their needed oxygen

Zinc—oversees body processes and aids in brain function

Magnesium—necessary for nerve functioning, known as known as the antistress mineral

Calcium—makes you less jumpy, more relaxed

227. Other Drugs Can Add to Your Problems

Alcohol is a nerve depressant. If you take tranquilizers and a drink, the combination of the two can cause a severe depression—or even death.

If you're on the pill and depressed,
it's not surprising.

If you take Darvon with a tranquilizer, you might find yourself experiencing tremors and mental confusion. The same thing can happen if you combine a sedative with an antihistamine (such as any found in over-the-counter cold preparations).

Oral contraceptives deplete the body of B_6, B_{12}, folic acid, and vitamin C. If you're on the pill and depressed, it is not surprising. Your need for B_6, necessary for normal tryptophan metabolism, is fifty to a hundred times a non–pill user's requirement.

DRUGS THAT YOU MIGHT NOT THINK WOULD CAUSE DEPRESSION—BUT CAN

- Adrenocorticoids
- Baclofen (Lioresal)
- Beta-blockers (Inderal)
- Antihypertensives
- Estrogens
- Antiarthritis medicines
- Potassium supplements
- Procainamide
- Propoxyphene (Darvon)
- Any sex hormones
- Trimethobenzamide (Tigan)

228. Any Questions About Chapter XV?

Every once in a while I find myself depressed when there's really nothing in my life to be depressed about. I'm a twenty-nine-year-old male, happily married, and I don't know why I go into these depressions. Could there be a dietary reason?

Absolutely! Especially if you're consoling yourself with sugar-rich foods. Sugar, be it in refined carbohydrates, alcohol, or whatever, can deplete your body of B vitamins, especially vitamin B_1, which can bring on depression. Amino acids (see sections 75–82) such as tyrosine, tryptophan, and phenylanine can all be used as antidepressants. Check with your doctor, but I'd recommend 500–2,000 mg. (2 g.) of a combination of these amino acids, taken at bedtime or in the morning, with water or juice (no protein).

XVI
Drugs and You

229. Let's Start with Caffeine

There are no doubts about it, caffeine is a powerful drug. That's right, *drug*. Chances are you're not just enjoying your daily coffees or colas, you're addicted to them.

> Caffeine is the most psychoactive
> drug in the world.

Caffeine acts directly upon the central nervous system. It brings about an almost immediate sense of clearer thought and lessens fatigue. It also stimulates the release of stored sugar from the liver, which accounts for the "lift" coffee, cola, and chocolate (the caffeine big three) give. But these benefits may be far outweighed by the side effects:

• The release of stored sugar places heavy stress on the endocrine system.
• Heavy coffee drinkers often develop nervousness or become jittery.
• Coffee-drinking housewives demonstrated symptoms

typical of drug withdrawal when switched to a decaffeinated beverage.

• Dr. John Minton, professor of surgery at Ohio State University and specialist in cancer oncology, has found that excessive intake of methylxanthines (active chemicals in caffeine) can cause benign breast disease and prostate problems.

• Caffeine can rob the body of B vitamins, especially inositol, as well as vitamin C, zinc, potassium, and other minerals.

• Coffee increases the acidity in your gastrointestinal tract and can cause rectal itching.

• Many doctors consider caffeine a culprit in hypertensive heart disease.

• The British medical journal *Lancet* reported a strong relationship between coffee consumption and cancer of the bladder and the lower urinary tract.

• People who drink five cups of coffee daily have a 50 percent greater chance of having heart attacks than non–coffee drinkers.

• The *Journal of the American Medical Association* reports a disease called caffeinism, with symptoms of appetite loss, weight loss, irritability, insomnia, feelings of flushing, chills, and sometimes a low fever.

• Caffeine has been shown to interfere with DNA replication.

• The Center for Science in the Public Interest advises pregnant women to stay away from caffeine, since studies have shown that the amount contained in about four cups of coffee per day causes birth defects in test animals.

• High doses of caffeine will cause laboratory animals to go into convulsions and then die.

Caffeine can be highly toxic (the lethal dose estimated to be around 10 g.). New research shows that one quart of coffee consumed in three hours can destroy much of the body's thiamine.

230. You're Getting More than You Think

The following table shows the amount of caffeine (in milligrams) consumed in specific beverages and drugs:

BEVERAGE	12-OUNCE CAN OR BOTTLE
Coca-Cola	64.7 mg.
Dr. Pepper	60.9 mg.
Mr. Pibb	58.8 mg.
Mellow Yellow	52.8 mg.
Mountain Dew	54.7 mg.
Diet Dr. Pepper	54.2 mg.
Tab	49.4 mg.
Pepsi-Cola	43.1 mg.
Diet Pepsi/Pepsi Lite	36.0 mg.
R.C. Cola	33.7 mg.
Diet R.C.	33.0 mg.
Diet-Rite	31.7 mg.
Coffee	*Per Serving*
Instant	66.0 mg.
Percolated	110.0 mg.
Dripolated	146.0 mg.
Tea Bags	
Black 5-minute brew	46.0 mg.
Black 1-minute brew	28.0 mg.
Loose Tea	
Black 6-minute brew	40.0 mg.
Green 5-minute brew	35.0 mg.
Cocoa	13.0 mg.

DRUGS	PER PILL
Anacin	32.0 mg.

DRUGS	PER PILL
Bio Slim T capsules	140.0 mg.
Cafergot	100.0 mg.
Dexatrim	200.0 mg.
Empirin	32.0 mg.
Emprazil	30.0 mg.
Excedrin	65.0 mg.
(Excedrin PM has no caffeine but does have an antihistamine.)	
Florinal	130.0 mg.
Midol	32.4 mg.
No Doz	100.0 mg.
Soma Compound	32.0 mg.
Triaminicin	30.0 mg.
Vanquish	33.0 mg.
Vivarin	200.0 mg.

231. Caffeine Alternatives

Decaffeinated coffee is *not* the best solution to the caffeine problem. Trichloroethylene, which was first used to remove caffeine, was found to cause a high incidence of cancer in test animals. Though the manufacturers have switched to methylene chloride, which is safer, it, too, introduces the same carbon-to-chlorine bond into the body that is characteristic of so many toxic insecticides.

> Ginseng can give you a
> real lift.

Regular tea is not the answer, either, since that has nearly as much caffeine. But herb teas can be quite invigorating, and most natural-food stores have a wide variety to choose from. Then, too, ginseng can give you a real lift, much like the one you get from caffeine, without the side effects.

Colas, diet or regular, have become as popular as coffee for those who enjoy the caffeine boost. Try substituting club soda or mineral water, or even a flavored soda if you must. You won't get the caffeine lift, but you'll be doing your body a big favor.

232. What Alcohol Does to Your Body

Alcohol is the most widely used drug in our society, and because it is so available, most people don't think of it as a drug. But it is; and if misused, it can cause a lot of damage to your body.

• Alcohol is not a stimulant, but actually a sedative-depressant of the central nervous system.
• It is capable of rupturing veins.
• It does not warm you up, but causes you to feel colder by increasing perspiration and body heat loss.
• It destroys brain cells by causing the withdrawal of necessary water from them.
• It can deplete the body of vitamins B_1, B_2, B_6, B_{12}, folic acid, vitamin C, vitamin K, zinc, magnesium, and potassium.
• Four drinks a day are capable of causing organ damage.
• It can hamper the liver's ability to process fat.

233. What You Drink and When You Drink It

Just because the alcohol content varies in different beverages, don't be fooled. It is true that beer has only about 4 percent alcohol, wine about 12 percent, and whiskey up to 50 percent; but a can of beer, a glass of wine, and a shot of whiskey all have virtually the identical inebriation potential. In other words, four cans of beer can get you just as tipsy as four shots of tequila.

> A Bloody Mary at breakfast is
> more harmful than a whiskey
> sour at dinner.

Surprisingly, what you drink doesn't matter nearly as much as *when* you drink it. Dr. John D. Palmer, of the University of Massachusetts, reports that the length of time alcohol remains circulating in your blood varies throughout the day. This means, of course, that the more time the alcohol spends in your blood, the more time it has to act on your brain cells. Between 2 A.M. and noon are the most vulnerable hours, while late afternoon to early evening are the least. A cocktail at dinner will be burned away 25 percent faster than a Bloody Mary at breakfast, and the last drink of a party, consumed after midnight, is metabolized relatively more slowly than the ones that preceded it, producing a more lasting rise in blood alcohol.

234. Vitamins to Decrease Your Taste for Alcohol

> Heavy drinkers can break
> the habit.

Research at the University of Texas has shown that if alcoholic mice are fed nutritious, vitamin-enriched diets, they quickly lose their interest in alcohol. This seems to hold true for people, since heavy drinkers have been able to break the habit—and even lose interest—with the right diet and proper nutritional supplements. Vitamins A, D, E, C, and all the B vitamins—especially B_{12}, B_6, and B_1—along with choline, inositol, niacin, and a very high-protein diet have brought about the best results. Dr. H. L. Newbold, of New York, who has worked with alcoholics, recommends building up to 5 glutamine capsules (200 mg.)—*not glutamic acid*—three times a day to control drinking and working with a good nutritionally oriented doctor for the best all-around regimen (see section 278).

In experiments done by the Veterans' Administration, a supplement of tryptophan, given in larger concentrations than occur in a normal diet, has helped alcoholics achieve normal sleeping patterns by reducing or normalizing the fragmentation of dreaming (REM). Because serotonin, a natural tranquilizer substance in the brain, has been shown to be reduced in alcoholism, tryptophan (500 mg. to 3 g. at bedtime is recommended) can help alcoholics stay dry by relieving some of the symptoms of alcohol-related body chemistry disorders.

235. The Lowdown on Marijuana and Hashish

Marijuana and hashish come from the hemp plant *Cannabis sativa*. The marijuana consists of the chopped leaves and stems of the plant, while the hashish is formed from the resin scraped from the flowering tops.

Both of these drugs can be either smoked or eaten. If smoked, the effects usually last from one to three hours. If eaten, they can last from four to ten hours, though it takes longer for the user to feel them.

Unlike other illicit drugs, marijuana and hashish have the unusual property of "reverse tolerance," meaning that seasoned users need less of the drug to get high than first-timers. Essentially, these drugs act as intoxicants, relaxants, tranquilizers, appetite stimulants, and mild hallucinogens, though effects vary with the individual.

The smoking of one joint can cause a rise in blood pressure, an increased heartbeat, a lowering of body temperature and vitamin C levels in the blood. It has been found, too, that smoking marijuana during pregnancy can cause low birth weight in newborns and increase the risk of lung cancer.

CAUTION: Toxic psychosis can occur if *Cannabis* is eaten and the user hasn't been able to judge the amount ingested.

Supplements and Foods That Can Help Users

Increase your intake of citrus fruits and green leafy vegetables. (Those "munchies" usually give you more than your share of refined sugars and carbohydrates, meaning that you've deprived yourself of necessary B vitamins.)

Vitamin C (time release), 1,000 mg. A.M. and P.M.

Vitamin E, 100–400 IU 1 to 3 times daily to protect your lungs

236. Cocaine Costs a Lot More than You Think—In More Ways than One

Cocaine is a vasoconstrictor, a stimulant of the central nervous system, and potentiates the effects of nerve stimulation. Applied externally, it blocks nerve impulses and produces a numbing sensation.

> The wrong "cut" can kill.

What users get—no matter how much they pay—is rarely more than 60 percent pure cocaine. The rest is the "cut," which is used by dealers to dilute or enhance the drug for more profit. Some cuts are relatively harmless: lactose, dextrose, inositol (a B vitamin), and mannitol. Other nondrug cuts such as cornstarch, talcum powder, and flour can be dangerous because they are basically insoluble in blood and can clot up in the body. *Benzocaine,* which is pharmacologically active, can also cause blood clots and serious complications when used as a cut for cocaine.

Because the drug is absorbed rapidly through the mucous membranes, nasal inhalation is the most popular form of taking cocaine, though it is also often applied locally under the tongue and eyelids, and on the genital region. It can also be injected intravenously or smoked in a process called "free basing."

The short-lived effects of coke (about one-half hour) are usually euphoria, and feelings of psychic energy and self-confidence, but then more of the drug is necessary to recapture the high. Psychological dependence is strong.

Aside from causing nosebleeds, rapid heartbeat, cold sweats, and in some cases the feeling that gnats or bugs are crawling on you, cocaine can cause convulsions, vomiting, and even anaphylactic shock. The biggest danger is that its toxicity is unpredictable, because even small doses with the wrong cut can cause serious problems. Immediate death can result from cocaine poisoning, usually caused by too rapid absorption of the drug through intravenous injection.

Supplements and Foods to Help Users
High-potency multiple vitamin and mineral A.M. and P.M.

High-potency multiple mineral A.M. and P.M.
Vitamin C, 1,000 mg., vitamin E, 200–400 IU, and
  vitamin B complex, 100 mg., all 1–3 times daily

237. Help for Coming Down or Kicking the Cocaine Habit

Tyrosine, an amino acid that's usually found in meat
and wheat (see section 82), has been found to alleviate
the depression, fatigue, and irritability that make quit-
ting cocaine so difficult. At Fair Oaks Hospital in
Summit, New Jersey, addicts took the amino acid in
their orange juice for twelve days. They also took
vitamin C, the B vitamins (thiamine, niacin, and
riboflavin), and tyrosine hydroxylase, the enzyme that
helps the body use tyrosine. The results were remarkably effective; in addicts, depression declined 70 percent.

238. Whether ℞ or Over the Counter, There Are Alternatives to Drugs

Americans consume over 1.5 million pounds of tranquilizers, more than 800,000 pounds of barbiturates,
and well over 4 million pounds of antibiotics a year.
Are all these drugs necessary? Probably not; but when
people pay for a visit to their doctor, they expect to
walk away with a prescription.

  But there are alternatives, which orthomolecular physicians and nutritionally minded individuals are trying
before resorting to drugs.

Inositol and pantothenic acid
instead of sleeping pills

Dr. Robert C. Atkins, author of *Dr. Atkins' Diet Revolution*, has his patients try pantothenic acid and about 2,000 mg. of inositol as sleep-inducers, instead of Seconal, Nembutal, Butisol, or other barbiturate sleeping pills.

So before you pop that next pill, you might want to consider some natural alternatives.

DRUG	NATURAL ALTERANTIVES
Antacids	Papaya and multiple digestive enzymes
Antibiotics and antihistamines	Garlic, vitamin C, and (yep, it's true) chicken soup have amazing antibiotic and antihistamine properties. Other fine infection fighters are vitamin A, pantothenic acid, and folic acid.
Antidepressants	Choline, calcium, and magnesium; vitamins B_1, B_6, and B_{12}, L-tryptophan and L-phenylalanine
Antidiarrhesis	Carrots, niacin, and lactobacillus acidophilus yogurt for diarrhea caused by antibiotics
Antinauseants	Vitamins B_1 and B_6 can help alleviate nausea due to motion or morning sickness. Niacin and vitamin P can help in the treatment of dizziness and queasiness due to diseases of the inner ear.
Decongestants	Vitamins A, C, P, garlic, and potassium
Diuretics (water pills)	Alfalfa and vitamin B_6 can work as natural diuretics.
Laxatives	Vitamin C, vitamins B_1, B_2, B_6, and B_{12}, potassium, acidophilus, alfalfa, bran, and water
Tranquilizers (sedatives, relaxants, and the like)	Choline, vitamins B_1, B_6, B_{12}, niacin, calcium, and magnesium; manganese, zinc, pantothenic acid and inositol, and L-tryptophan

239. The Great Medicine Rip-Off

More than ever before, Americans are gulping down drugs. What most people don't realize is that a lot of these medications—prescription as well as over the counter—are taking as much as they're giving, at least nutritionally. All too often the drugs either stop the absorption of nutrients or interfere with the cells' ability to use them.

A recent study showed that ingredients found in common over-the-counter cold, pain, and allergy remedies actually lowered the blood level of vitamin A. Since vitamin A protects and strengthens the mucous membranes lining the nose, throat, and lungs, a deficiency could give bacteria a cozy home to multiply in, prolonging the illness the drug was meant to alleviate.

> Aspirin can *triple* the excretion
> rate of vitamin C.

Aspirin, the household wonder drug, the most common ingredient in pain relievers, cold and sinus remedies, is a vitamin-C thief. Even a small amount can *triple* the excretion rate of vitamin C from the body. It can also lead to a deficiency of folic acid and vitamin B, which could cause anemia as well as digestive disturbances.

Corticosteroids (cortisone, prednisone), used for easing arthritis pain, skin problems, blood and eye disorders, and asthma, have been found to be related to lowered zinc levels.

According to a study that appeared in the *Postgraduate Medical Journal,* a significant number of people who take barbiturates have low calcium levels.

Laxatives and antacids, taken by millions, have been

found to disturb the body's calcium and phosphorus metabolism. And any laxative taken to excess can deplete large amounts of potassium.

Diuretics, commonly prescribed for high blood pressure, and antibiotics are also potassium thieves.

The following is a list of drugs that induce vitamin deficiencies and the vitamins they deplete. Look it over before you take your next medicine.

THIEVING DRUG	NUTRIENTS DEPLETED
Alcohol (including alcohol-containing cough syrups, elixirs, and OTC medications such as Nyquil)	Vitamins A, B_1, B_2, biotin, choline, niacin, vitamin B_{15}, folic acid, and magnesium
Ammonium Chloride (e.g., Ambenyl Expectorant, Triaminicol Decongestant Cough Syrup, P.V. Tussin Syrup)	Vitamin C
Antacids (e.g., Maalox, Mylanta, Gelusil, Tums, Rolaids)	B complex and vitamin A
Anticoagulants (e.g., Coumadin, Dicumarol, Panwarfin)	Vitamins A and K
Antihistamines (e.g., Chlor-Trimeton, Pyribenzamine)	Vitamin C
Aspirin (and remember, APC drugs contain *aspirin*)	Vitamins A, B complex, C; calcium, potassium
Barbiturates (e.g., Phenobarbital, Seconal, Nembutal, Butisol, Tuinal)	Vitamins A, D, folic acid, and C
Caffeine (present in all APC medicines)	B_1, inositol and biotin; potassium, zinc; can also inhibit calcium and iron assimilation
Chloramphenicol (Chloromycetin)	Vitamin K and niacin
Clofibrate (Atromid-S)	Vitamin K
Colchicine (ColBENEMID)	B_{12}, A, and potassium
Diethylstilbestrol (DES)	Vitamin B_6
Diuretics (e.g., Diuril, Hydro-DIURIL, Ser-Ap-Es, Lasix)	B complex, potassium, magnesium, and zinc
Fluorides	Vitamin C

THIEVING DRUG	NUTRIENTS DEPLETED
Glutethimide (Doriden)	Folic acid
Indomethacin (Indocin)	Vitamins B₁ and C
Isoniazid (Inh, Nydrazid)	B₆
Kanamycin (Kantrex)	Vitamins K and B₁₂
Laxatives, lubricant (e.g., castor oil, mineral oil)	Vitamins A, D, E, K, calcium, and phosphorus
Meprednisone (Betapar)	Vitamins B₆, C, zinc, and potassium
Methotrexate (Mexate)	Folic acid
Nitrofurantoin (e.g., Furadantin, Macrodantin)	Folic acid
Oral contraceptives (e.g., Brevicon, Demulen, Enovid, Lo/Ovral, Norinyl, Ovral)	Folic acid, vitamins C, B₂, B₆, B₁₂, and E
Penicillamine (Cuprimine)	Vitamin B₆
Penicillin (in all its forms)	Vitamins B₆, niacin, and K
Phenylbutazone (e.g., Azolid, Butazolidin)	Folic acid
Phenytoin (Dilantin)	Folic acid and vitamin D
Prednisone (e.g., Meticorten, Prednisolone, Orasone)	Vitamins B₆, D, C, zinc, and potassium
Propantheline (Pro-Banthine)	Vitamin K
Pyrimethamine (Daraprim)	Folic acid
Sulfonamides, systemic (e.g., Bactrim, Gantanol, Tantrisin, Septra)	Folic acid, vitamins K and B₂
Sulfonamides and topical steroids (e.g., Aerosporin, Cortisporin, Neosporin, Polysporin)	Vitamins K, B₁₂, and folic acid
Tetracyclines (e.g., Achromhycin V, Sumycin, Tetracyn)	Vitamin K, calcium, magnesium, and iron
Tobacco	Vitamins C, B₁, and folic acid; calcium
Triamterene (Dyrenium)	Folic acid
Trifluoperazine (Stelazine)	Vitamin B₁₂

240. Any Questions About Chapter XVI?

I know that coffee can give you the jitters, but I've switched to drinking decaffeinated and still find myself getting moody and uptight. Can such a small amount of caffeine do this?

Caffeine isn't the only substance in coffee that has an effect on behavior. There is, though not yet identified, another substance in both regular and decaffeinated coffee (but not in tea) that blocks the normal activity of brain opiates (endorphins), which act as painkillers and mood elevators.

Some prescription medications that I take are specifically labeled "Do not drink alcoholic beverages while taking this medication." If there is no label, does that mean it's safe to have a drink while on them?

Only if you think that Russian roulette is safe. Alcohol can interact adversely with almost all drugs. In fact, any drug that's available in time-release or spansule form can become dangerous if taken in conjunction with alcohol. The coating that's supposed to allow the drug to be released slowly over an extended time period (usually eight to twelve hours) can dissolve rapidly in alcohol and give you an uncomfortable and potentially toxic dose of the medication. My advice is get well first, then celebrate afterward.

What is the pharmacological or physiological reason for the "down" that seems to follow even moderate cocaine use?

It's primarily caused by the depletion of the body's stores of dopamine and norepinephrine. These are chemicals that the brain normally uses to relay energy messages. The high from cocaine comes from exciting these neurotransmitters, while at the same time inhibiting serotonin, the chemical that can calm you down. So while a cocaine user is "up," the brain surges at a breakneck pace, and then when the neurotransmitters are depleted, the user crashes, which sets up a desire for more of the drug. (See section 237 for a good animo acid antidote.)

XVII

Losing It—Diets by the Pound

241. The Atkins Diet

This diet ignores calorie content and focuses on carbohydrate restriction; but unlike other low-carbohydrate programs, Dr. Atkins' calls for *no* carbohydrates (at least for the first week). By doing this, the body begins to throw off ketones (tiny carbon fragments that are by-products of incompletely burned fat) in amounts sufficient to account for substantial weight loss. According to Dr. Atkins, because carbohydrates are the first fuel your body burns for energy, if none are taken in, then the body will draw upon stored fat for fuel. And as ketones are excreted, hunger as well as weight will disappear.

The pros and cons are many, but if you are on this diet, Dr. Atkins recommends a high-potency vitamin supplement. I would suggest following the MVP program outlined in section 128 and taking an additional 1,000 mg. vitamin C with bioflavonoids if you've cut out all citrus fruit. Also take at least 50 mg. B complex with the morning and evening meal, 1 g. potassium divided over three meals, and 400 to 800 mcg. folic acid daily.

242. The Stillman Diet

Dr. Irwin Stillman's Quick Weight Loss Diet, often called "The Water Diet" because it requires drinking eight glasses of water daily, is essentially an all-protein program—no fats or carbohydrates. It permits no vegetables or fruits, no dairy products or grains, and is said to burn up about 275 more calories daily than a diet that contains the same number of calories but includes other elements, such as carbohydrates and fats. You don't count calories, but you're not supposed to stuff yourself, either, and the average weight loss is said to be between five and fifteen pounds per week.

Even Dr. Stillman recognized the need for supplementation while on his diet. He recommended a multivitamin-mineral tablet for anyone following his regimen and a high-potency multivitamin-mineral tablet for anyone on it who is over forty or eating very small amounts of food.

My own feeling is that anyone on Dr. Stillman's all-protein regimen should be taking a high-potency vitamin and chelated mineral tablet twice daily, along with 1,000 mg. vitamin C complex (time release) and a high-potency multiple chelated mineral tablet. Also, because the heavy water intake tends to flush the B vitamins as well as C from the body more quickly, a time-release vitamin B complex would be advisable, as would 400 to 800 mcg. folic acid and 1 g. potassium divided over three meals.

243. The Scarsdale Diet

This fourteen-day crash diet, on which you can lose up to twenty pounds, was created by Dr. Herman Tarnower and made famous in his book *The Complete Scarsdale Medical Diet* (Rawson, Wade Publishers, Inc.). It is basically a variation on the low-calorie, low-fat, low-carbohydrate, high-protein regimen. The difference between the Scarsdale Diet and the Stillman and Atkins diets is that Dr. Tarnower has added a no-decision factor to his plan. In other words, you eat exactly what's on the menu for each meal every day. And no switching, at least not for two weeks.

Taking all responsibility from the dieter—except that of following instructions—has made the Scarsdale a popular and effective regimen.

As with any diet, because of the sudden cut in food intake, supplements are advised. A basic MVP (see section 128) should be taken if you're on the Scarsdale. Also recommended are vitamin E (dry form), 200 to 400 IU daily, and a good B complex.

244. Weight Watchers

This is a long-term regimen that advocates three meals a day with measured portions of protein, carbohydrates, and fat.

Though the program is nutritionally well rounded, most Weight Watchers I've met agree that supplements have helped them keep up their energy levels while their calorie intake goes down. A multivitamin-mineral tablet, a multiple chelated mineral, and a vitamin C complex, 500 to 1,000 mg., taken one to two times daily should fill the bill.

245. The Drinking Man's Diet

This is another low-carbohydrate, high-fat and high-protein diet, but with the added appeal of allowing alcohol to be part of the regimen. Allegedly based on the U.S. air Force diet (though the Air Force denies it), this one advocates keeping your carbohydrate count to 60 g. a day.

The diet states specifically that it is for healthy people and cautions adherents to get at least 30 g. of carbohydrates daily and enough vitamin C.

Anyone on this diet would be well advised to take a vitamin-C supplement, along with a general MVP (see section 128) regimen, and B complex three times a day because of the alcohol.

246. Liquid Protein and Cambridge Diets

These diets are dangerous and potentially lethal. (The liquid protein diet is no longer on the market.)

The Cambridge Diet offers three liquid *allegedly* "nutritionally balanced" meals a day totaling 330 calories, which is an intake that can be aligned to semistarvation. Dr. Sami Hashim, a world-renowned expert in the treatment of obesity, has stated that "anyone who is on a diet of 600 calories or less should be in the hospital."

Radical diets such as these can cause abnormal heart function and severe deficiencies in vital minerals due to extremely rapid weight loss. I couldn't in good conscience offer supplement suggestions, since I firmly believe that these diets should not be undertaken without strict medical supervision.

247. Zen Macrobiotic Diet

Contrary to popular belief, this diet is not connected with the Zen Buddhists but is the creation of a Japanese man named George Ohsawa. Though it has gained many adherents, it is nutritionally dangerous when strictly followed.

There are ten stages to the diet, and milk is prohibited. You start by giving up dessert and work backward until you're in the highest stage and eating nothing but grains, preferably brown rice. The diet, based on the Oriental yin/yang philosophy, restricts fluid intake, which is dangerous, as is the lack of nutrients provided in meals consisting of nothing but brown rice. Followers believe that if your thoughts are right, you can produce vitamins, minerals, and proteins within your own body and actually change one element to another.

Just in case your thoughts aren't always right, it would be advisable, if you are on this diet or just a strict vegetarian one, to take supplements. A high-potency vegetarian multivitamin-mineral tablet twice daily along with a good B complex with folic acid is recommended. Also take vitamin B_{12}, 100 mcg., one to three times a day.

248. Fructose Diet

This fourteen-day diet is for people who crave sweets. The secret is a supplement of fructose, a natural sugar, that not only satisfies your hunger and keeps up your energy, but allows you to lose a pound a day.

Developed by Dr. J. T. Cooper, the fructose diet is basically a low-calorie program, but by taking 36 to 42 g. of fructose a day you are supposed to lose your craving for food. Unlike other dietary sugars, fructose doesn't require insulin to enter the body's cells. It is absorbed directly, eliminating the hypoglycemic (low blood sugar) reaction brought on by excess insulin, which is what makes dieters feel hungry.

Fructose is obtained from vegetables such as artichokes and corn. It is available in powder, flavored 2-g. chewable tablets, and syrup.

Ten glasses of water daily are recommended along with supplements. An MVP (see section 128) is important, as is potassium, 99 mg. (elemental) taken three times a day—one tablet with each meal.

249. Kelp, Lecithin, Vinegar, B₆ Diet

This low-profile but effective diet has been around for more than a decade and still seems to be popular. The basic components of the diet can be obtained in one tablet that contains kelp, lecithin, apple cider vinegar, and vitamin B₆, There are two potencies available: single and double strength. (With the single strength you take two tablets with each meal and with the double strength you take one.)

As with any diet that cuts down caloric intake, a good multivitamin-mineral tablet taken with breakfast and dinner is recommended. Also take a B complex and 1,000 mg. vitamin C (time release) twice daily.

250. Mindell Dieting Tips

• Before starting any diet, check with your physician. If you don't feel that your family doctor understands your dieting needs, contact a bariatrician, who specializes in the field. For the name of one in your area, write to the

American Society of Bariatric Physicians, Suite 300, 5200 South Quebec, Englewood, Colorado 80111. (Enclose a stamped self-addressed envelope.)

• If you're on a low- or no-carbohydrate diet, beware of artificially sweetened "sugarless" or "dietetic" gum or candy that has sorbitols, mannitols, or hexitols. These ingredients are metabolized in the system as carbohydrates, only more slowly.

• If you're on a diet that allows alcohol, a glass of wine before dinner stimulates the gastric juices and aids in proper digestion.

• Watch out for these diet fallacies:

Gelatin dessert is nonfattening.
Grapefruit causes you to lose weight.
Fruits have no calories.
High-protein foods have no calories.
A pound of steak is not as fattening as a potato.
Toast has much fewer calories than bread.

• Whatever you're eating, sit down to eat it, and eat it slowly. (You might expend more calories standing than sitting, but you tend to eat more that way, too.) Also, don't read or watch TV until you finish your meal.

• When selecting fruit, remember that all fruits are not equal, that an apple, a banana, or a pear has more calories and carbohydrates than half a cantaloupe, a cup of raw strawberries, or a fresh tangerine.

• When choosing your vegetable, take green beans instead of peas (you save 41 calories on a half-cup serving), spinach instead of mixed vegetables (you save 35 calories), and mashed potatoes—if you must—instead of hashed browns (you save 139 calories).

• Carbohydrate watchers, don't underestimate onions; one cup of cooked onions has 18 g.

• If you're counting every calorie, realize that one tablespoon of lecithin granules contains 50 calories and a lecithin capsule about 8.

• Try a one-day-a-week water fast (the ancient Greeks did it). Limit yourself to cold tap water (not iced) or herb tea with lemon or lime juice. Nothing else. This should pep you up, too.

251. Mindell Vitamin-Balanced Diet to Lose and Live By

I know your mother told it to you, but it is true anyway—breakfast *is* the most important meal of the day. It comes after the longest period of time that you've been without food, and you cannot catch up nutritionally by eating a good lunch or dinner later.

If you're dieting, it is especially important to perk up your energy level at the start of the day.

BREAKFAST

8 oz. nonfat or low-fat milk (or juice)

A flavored low-calorie protein powder that contains nutritional yeast, lecithin, and fructose

4 ice cubes

Mix well in blender for 60 seconds. Calories approximately: 150

This mixture can be frozen and used as a dessert for dinner or a pick-me-up snack, if your calories quotient allows.

Lunch is a tricky meal. Fast-food restaurants are seductively convenient, and nothing blows a diet faster than "a few French fries" and a "tiny milkshake." If you really want to lose weight, think more along these lines:

LUNCH
Monday, Wednesday, Saturday, and Sunday
A modest portion (3–5 ounces) of water-packed canned or fresh fish, a large raw vegetable salad (with lemon or vinegar dressing), and a piece of fruit.

Tuesday, Thursday, and Friday
2 eggs (prepared without fat) or cottage or pot cheese (no more than 1 cup), raw vegetables, 1 slice of bread with a light coating of margarine, and a fruit for dessert. (The American Heart Association suggests only 3 whole eggs per week, though many doctors allow more. Check with your own physician.)

Dinner is usually a dieter's downfall, but it doesn't have to be that way:

DINNER
Five nights a week you should have fish (sole, trout, salmon, halibut, and the like) or poultry broiled, boiled, or roasted (remove skin before eating poultry); and two nights a week you can have meat, once again broiled, boiled, or roasted; a cooked vegetable, a large salad (no more than a teaspoon of oil in the dressing), a small boiled or baked potato once or twice a week, and a fresh fruit for dessert.

Stay away from alcohol—try sparkling mineral water with lime instead. As for other beverages, herb teas and plain old water are best.

Take your supplements six days a week and rest on the seventh. By doing this, you'll never have to worry about a buildup of fat-soluble vitamins in the system.

SUPPLEMENTS

Time-release multiple vitamin with chelated minerals (at least 50 mg. B_1, B_2, and B_6 per tablet) taken A.M. and P.M.

Time-release vitamin C, 1,000 mg. with rose hips bioflavonoids, 2 tablets taken A.M. and P.M.

A multiple chelated mineral tablet with at least 500 mg. calcium and 250 mg. magnesium per tablet (must also have manganese, zinc, iron, selenium, chromium, copper, iodine, and potassium) taken A.M. and P.M.

Dry vitamin E, 400 IU—D-alpha-tocopherol with selenium, chromium, vitamin C, and ascorbates taken A.M. and P.M.

RNA 100 mg.—DNA 100 mg., 3 tablets daily, 6 days a week

SOD (see section 266), 125 mcg. daily, 6 days a week

DHEA (see section 266), 3 tablets daily, 1 hour before meals

Lecithin, 1,200 mg. (6 capsules) daily (If you use lecithin granules in breakfast drink, this supplement is not necessary.)

252. Any Questions About Chapter XVII?

I was on the Cambridge Diet for four weeks, lost 25 pounds, and felt fine. Why is it considered so dangerous?

Because it is (see section 246), and you were lucky. Many times dieters suffer heart failure when they go off semistarvation diets and resume normal eating because of the radical shifts in body salts and water. Additionally, diets such as the Cambridge formula do not teach you how to change your eating habits and keep off the weight you lose . . . in fact, most people regain at least half the weight they've lost within two years.

XVIII

So You Think You Don't Eat Much Sugar and Salt

253. Kinds of Sugars

More than a hundred substances that qualify as sweet can be called sugars. The ones we come in contact with most often are *fructose*, a natural sugar found in fruit and honey; *glucose*, the body's blood sugar and the simplest form of sugar in which a carbohydrate is assimilated; *dextrose*, made from cornstarch and chemically identical to glucose; *lactose*, milk sugar; *maltose*, the sugar formed from the starch by the action of yeast; and *sucrose*, the sugar that is obtained from sugar cane or beets and refined to the product that reaches us as granules.

> Brown sugar is merely sugar crystals
> coated with molasses syrup.

Brown sugar, which many people assume to be healthier than white sugar, is merely sugar crystals coated with molasses syrup. (In the United States most brown sugar is made by simply spraying refined white sugar with the molasses syrup.) Raw sugar is banned in the United States because it contains contaminants. When it's partially refined and cleaned up, it can be sold as turbinado sugar. Honey is a blend of fructose and glucose. Then there are the various corn sweeteners, derived from cornstarch and composed mainly of dextrose, maltose, and the more complex sugars.

254. Dangers of Too Much Sugar

Ketchup has 8 percent more sugar
than ice cream.

The big problem with sugar is that we eat too much of it (over 154 pounds per person in 1984) and often don't even know it. All carbohydrate sweeteners qualify as sugar, even though they may be called by other names; and when sucrose is the number-three ingredient on a box of cereal, corn syrup number five, and honey number seven, you don't realize it but you're eating something that is 50 percent sugar!

The consumer today is hooked on sugar right from the start. Baby formulas are frequently sweetened with sugar, as are many baby foods. Because sugar also acts as a preservative, retains and absorbs moisture, it's often in products we never think of as containing it, products such as salt, peanut butter, canned vegetables, bouillon cubes, and more. Would you believe that the ketchup you put on your hamburger has just less than 8 percent more sugar than ice cream? That cream substitute for coffee is 65 percent sugar compared to 51 percent for a chocolate bar?

The fact is, we're eating too much sugar for our

health. It is beyond argument that sugar is a prime factor in tooth decay. Also, one-third of our population is overweight, and obesity increases the possibility of heart disease, diabetes, hypertension, gallstones, back problems, and arthritis. Not that sugar alone is the cause, but its presence in foods induces you to eat more, and if you cut your calorie count without cutting your sugar intake, you'll lose nutrients faster than pounds. Sugar is also the villain where hypoglycemia is concerned and, though there have been arguments pro and con, directly or indirectly a factor in diabetes and heart disease.

255. How Sweet It Is

Hidden sugars are where you least expect them. If you want to be a sugar detective, my advice is to check labels. Look for sucrose substitutes such as corn syrup or corn sugar, and watch out for words ending in "-ose," which indicates the presence of sugar. A sugar by any name is still a sugar. And remember that not even medicines are immune from added sweeteners!

MEDICINES	SUGAR PER TABLESPOON
Alternagel Liquid	2,000 mg.
Basaljel Extra-strength Liquid	375 mg.
Gaviscon Liquid	1,500 mg.
Gaviscon-2 tablets	2,400 mg.
Maslox Plus tablets	575 mg.
Mylanta Liquid	2,000 mg.
Riopan Plus Chew Tablets	610 mg.

(When in doubt about sugar or saccharin content of any medication—ask your pharmacist.)

256. Dangers of Too Much Salt

Taking things with a grain of salt is all well and good, but eating things with it might be a different story. The normal intake of sodium chloride (table salt) is 6 to 18 g. daily, but an intake over 14 g. is considered excessive. And too many of us are being excessive. The average American consumes about 15 pounds (a bowling ball) of salt each year!

Too much salt can cause hypertension (high blood pressure), which increases the chances of heart disease, and has recently been cited as one of the causes for migraine headaches. It causes abnormal fluid retention, which can result in dizziness and swelling of the legs. It may also cause potassium to be lost in the urine. In addition, too much salt can harm you nutritionally by interfering with the proper utilization of protein foods.

257. High-Salt Traps

Just because you stay away from pretzels and snack foods and don't pour on the table salt doesn't mean you're not getting more salt than you should. Salt traps are as hidden from view as sugar ones.

If you want to keep your salt intake down:

• Hold back on beer. (There's 25 mg. sodium in every 12 ounces.)
• Avoid the use of baking soda, monosodium glutamate (MSG, Accent), and baking powder in food preparation.
• Stay away from laxatives, most of which contain sodium.
• Do not drink or cook with water treated by a home water softener; it adds sodium to the water.

• Look for the words SALT, SODIUM, or the chemical symbol *Na* when reading food labels.
• Don't eat cured meat such as ham, bacon, corned beef, or frankfurters, sausage, shellfish, any canned or frozen meat, poultry, or fish to which sodium has been added.
• When dining out, ask for an inside cut of meat, or chops or steaks without added salt.
• Watch out for diet sodas—the calories might be low, but the sodium content is *high!*

258. How Salty Is It?

APPROXIMATE SODIUM CONTENT OF COMMON FOODS

Item	Amount	Salt (mg.)
Pickle, dill	1 large	1,928
Frozen turkey three-course dinner (Swanson)	1 (17 oz.)	1,735
Soy Sauce	1 tbsp.	1,320
Pancakes (Hungry Jack Complete)	3 pancakes 4 in. each	1,150
Chicken noodle soup (Campbell's)	10 oz.	1,050
Tomato soup (Campbell's)	10 oz.	950
Green beans, canned (Del Monte)	1 cup	925
Cheese, pasteurized, processed American (Kraft)	2 oz.	890
Baked red kidney beans (B and M)	1 cup	810
Pizza, frozen (Celeste)	4 oz.	656
V8 vegetable juice	6 oz.	654
Danish cinnamon rolls w/raisins (Pillsbury)	1 serving	630
Pudding, instant chocolate (Jell-O)	½ cup	486
Bologna (Oscar Mayer)	2 slices	450
Tuna, in oil (Del Monte)	3 oz.	430
Frankfurter, beef (Oscar Mayer)	1	425

259. Any Questions About Chapter XVIII?

Isn't it true that in very hot weather you need salt supplements, especially if you do exercise and perspire heavily?

No! This is not only a myth, but one that could result in dangerous consequences. The truth is that salt tablets have a dehydrating effect and are never indicated. When you exercise, your body uses mechanisms to conserve salt—and since the average American eats somewhere around 60 or more times the salt that is needed by the body, salt depletion is highly unlikely. In fact, too much salt under those conditions can contribute to heat exhaustion and heat stroke. (In the very, *very* rare case where a salt deficiency might occur, replacement should be administered with a 0.1 percent solution of salt administered in drinking water—and a doctor should be consulted.)

I know that diet sodas are high in salt, but I've heard that plain club soda is, also. How much could it really have?

It could really have a lot—and it does! An 8-oz. glass of Canada Dry club soda has 75.0 mg.! You can get the same fizz from salt-free seltzer.

Is NutraSweet a safer artificial sweetener than saccharin?

I believe so. Unlike saccharin and cyclamate, Nutra-Sweet—or aspartame—has so far been found to be noncarcinogenic (cancer-causing). This is not to say that it's side-effect free. Since it is a combination of the amino acids L-aspartic acid and L-phenylalanine, the cautions that apply to those (see section 77) also apply to NutraSweet.

XIX

Staying Beautiful—Staying Handsome

260. Vitamins for Healthy Skin

What you look like on the outside depends a lot on what you do for yourself on the inside. And as far as your skin is concerned, vitamins and proper nutrition are essential.

To look your best, make sure you're getting 55 to 65 g. of protein a day. Drink eight glasses of water daily (herbal teas can count for a few of them), and keep your milk and yogurt consumption restricted to the nonfat variety. Keep away from chocolate, nuts, dried fruits, fried foods, cola drinks, coffee, alcohol, cigarettes, and excessive salt. Also, do not use sugar. Small amounts of honey or blackstrap molasses will sweeten just as well and you'll look better for it.

A good start toward healthy, glowing skin is a daily protein drink. It can be taken in place of any meal, but it makes an especially good breakfast.

PROTEIN DRINK

6 oz. nonfat milk
1 tbsp. nutritional yeast powder (lots of B vitamins)

3 tbsp. acidophilus (promotes friendly bacteria)

1 tbsp. granulated lecithin (breaks down bumps or cholesterol under the skin)

1 tbsp. protein powder

½–1 tbsp. blackstrap molasses or honey

Carob powder, bananas, strawberries, or any fresh fruit for flavoring

Mix in blender. (Add 3–4 ice cubes, if desired.)

SUPPLEMENTS

Multivitamin-mineral complex—1 daily

Take after any meal. Important for skin tone and nerve health.

B complex, 100 mg. (time release)—1 daily

Take after any meal. B_2 (riboflavin) and B_6 (pyridoxine) reduce facial oiliness and blackhead formation.

Vitamin A (dry form), 25,000 IU—2 daily for 5 days a week

Take 1 after breakfast and 1 after dinner. Maintains soft, smooth, disease-free skin. Builds resistance to infections.

Rose hips vitamin C, 1,000 mg. with bioflavonoids—3 daily

Take 1 after each meal and at bedtime. Aids in preventing the spread of acne. Promotes healing of wounds, bruising, and scar tissue. Helps to prevent breakage of capillaries on face.

Vitamin E (dry form), 400 IU—1–3 daily

Take 1 after each meal. Improves circulation in tiny face capillaries. Aids in healing by replacing cells on the skin's outer layer. Works with vitamin C in making skin less susceptible to acne. Use vitamin-E oil (28,000 IU per oz.) externally on skin for healing burns, abrasions, and scar tissue.

Multiple chelated minerals—6 daily

Take 2 tablets after each meal (or 3 in A.M. and P.M.). Helps maintain the acid-alkaline balance of the blood necessary for a clear complexion. Calcium is for soft, smooth skin tissue; copper for skin color; iron to improve pale skin; potassium for dry skin and acne; zinc for external and internal wound healing.

Choline and inositol, 1,000 mg. daily, after a large meal (Lecithin granules, 2 tbsp. daily, can be substituted for choline and inositol tabs.) Helps emulsify cholesterol (fatty deposits or bumps under the skin). Purifies the kidneys, which aids the skin.

Acidophilus—6 tbsp. daily

Take 2 tbsp. or 6 capsules after each meal. Helps fight skin eruptions caused by unfriendly bacteria in the system.

Chlorophyll—3 tsp. or 9 tablets daily

Take 1 tsp. or 3 tablets after each meal. Reduces hazard of bacterial contamination. Possesses antibiotic action. An excellent aid to wound healing, after washing thoroughly with a soap substitute made from the comfrey plant.

Cysteine, 1 g. daily

with 3 g. vitamin C

Take between meals with juice. Helps maintain supple, young-looking skin.

If face is badly blemished, extra zinc (chelated) is advised, 15–50 mg. daily. Aids in growth and repair of injured tissues.

261. Vitamins for Healthy Hair

Shampoos and conditioners are not enough. To make sure that you're giving your crowning glory its due, you have to be aware that nutrition plays a very important role in having terrific, shiny hair. Unlike the skin, hair cannot repair itself; but you *can* get new, healthier hair to grow.

The first thing to do is examine your diet. Does it include fish, wheat germ, yeast, and liver? It should. The vitamins and minerals that these foods supply are what your hair needs, along with frequent scalp massage, a good pH-balanced, protein-enriched shampoo, and supplements.

SUPPLEMENTS

Multivitamin-mineral complex—1 daily
Take after any meal. Important for general health of hair.

B complex, 100 mg. (time release)—1 daily
Take after any meal. B vitamins are essential for hair growth. Pantothenic acid, folic acid, and PABA help restore gray hair to its natural color.

Vitamin A, 10,000 IU—1–2 daily 5 days a week
Take A.M. and P.M. Works with vitamin B to keep hair shiny.

Cysteine, 1 g. daily with 3 g. vitamin C
Take between meals with juice. Hair is 10 to 14 percent cysteine, and this supplement can keep tresses looking lustrous.

Multiple chelated minerals—1 daily
Take with breakfast. Minerals such as silicon, sulfur, iodine, and iron help prevent falling hair.

Keep in mind that you need some fatty acids, vitamin B, and choline in your body for vitamin A to survive.

262. Vitamins for Hands and Feet

Your hands take lots of abuse. Detergents strip away natural oils, and water and weather alone can cause chapping. Rubber gloves are a good idea, but if you already have splits in your skin or some sort of dermatitis, they could *not* be put directly on your hands. (A pair of cotton gloves beneath the rubber ones will absorb perspiration and prevent reinfection.) Also, do not use cornstarch in the gloves; it can promote the growth of microorganisms. If you want to use something to absorb the moisture, try plain unscented talcum powder.

As for toenails and fingernails, the best remedy for problems is diet. Gelatin is commonly accepted as the cure for weak nails, but this is a misconception. The nails do need protein, but gelatin is a poor supplier. Not only are two essential amino acids missing, but another amino acid, glycine, is supplied in amounts you do not need. Foods rich in sulfur, such as egg yolks, should be part of your diet, and desiccated, defatted liver (tablets) should be taken as a supplement.

SUPPLEMENTS

Multivitamin-mineral complex—1 daily
   Take after any meal. Promotes general skin health and growth of nails.
B complex, 100 mg. (time release)—1 daily
   Take after any meal. Helps build resistance to fungus infections and vital to nail growth.
Vitamin A, 10,000 IU—1 daily 6 days a week
   Take after any meal. Helps to prevent splitting nails.

Vitamin E, 100–400 IU—1–2 daily
Take in A.M. and P.M. Necessary for proper utilization of vitamin A.

Multiple chelated minerals—1 daily
Take after any meal. Iron helps strengthen brittle nails, zinc gets rid of white spots.

263. Natural Cosmetics—What's in Them

Many cosmetics nowadays are advertised as "natural," but looking at the ingredients can cause you to wonder. To be sure of what you're getting, read the label carefully. The following explanations of cosmetic ingredients should make things clearer.

Amyl Dimethyl PABA—a sunscreening agent from PABA, a B-complex factor

Annatto—a vegetable color obtained from the seeds of a tropical plant

Avocado oil—a vegetable oil obtained from avocados

Caprylic/Capric triglyceride—an emollient obtained from coconut oil

Carrageenan—a natural thickening agent from dried Irish moss

Castor oil—an emollient oil collected from the pressing of castor bean seeds

Cetyl alcohol—a component of vegetable oils

Cetyl palmitate—a component of palm and coconut oils

Citric acid—a natural organic acid found widely in citrus plants

Cocamide DEA—a thickener obtained from coconut oil

Coconut oil—obtained by pressing the kernels of the seeds of the coconut palm

Decyl oleate—obtained from tallow or coconut oil

Disodium monolaneth-5-sulfosuccinate—obtained from lanolin and used to improve the texture of hair

Fragrance—oils obtained from flowers, grasses, roots, and stems that give off a pleasant or agreeable odor

Goat milk whey—protein-rich whey obtained from goat's milk

Glyceryl stearate—an organic emulsifier obtained from glycerin

Hydrogenated castor oil—a waxy material obtained from castor oil

Imidazolidinyl urea—a preservative derived naturally as a product of protein metabolism (hydrolysis)

Lanolin alcohol—a constituent of lanolin that performs as an emollient and emulsifier

Laureth-3—an organic material obtained from coconut and palm oils

Methyl glucoside sesquistearate—an organic emulsifier obtained from a natural simple sugar

Mineral oil—an organic emollient and lubricant

Olive oil—a natural oil obtained from olives

Peanut oil—a vegetable oil obtained from peanuts

Pectin—derived from citrus fruits and apple peel

PEG lanolin—an emollient and emulsifier obtained from lanolin

Petrolatum—petroleum jelly

P.O.E. (20) methyl glucoside sesquistearate—an organic emulsifier from a simple natural sugar

Potassium sorbate—obtained from sorbic acid found in the berries of mountain ash

Safflower oil-hybrid—a natural emollient obtained from a strain of specially cultivated plants

Sesame oil—oil of pressed sesame seeds

Sodium cetyl sulfate—a detergent and emulsifier obtained from coconut oil

Sodium laureth sulfate—a detergent obtained from coconut oil

Sodium lauryl sulfate—a detergent obtained from coconut oil

Sodium PCA—a natural-occurring humectant found in the skin where it acts as a natural moisturizer

Sorbic acid—a natural preservative derived from berries of mountain ash

Tocopherol—a natural vitamin E

Undecylenamide DEA—a natural preservative derived from castor oil

Water—the universal solvent, and the major constituent of all living material

264. Not So Pretty Drugs

Medications are necessary for certain conditions, but doctors often fail to mention their possible side effects. It is a rare physician who puts his patient on the pill and tells her that her face might break out or that she might suffer hair loss; but many women on oral contraceptives find this out soon enough. In fact, many drugs can be the cause of skin and other cosmetic problems. The following is a list of just a few:

Amytal	Skin rash, swollen eyelids, itchy skin
Butisol	Acne, pimples
Dalmane	Rash, flushes
Dexamyl	Swollen patches, itchy skin
Dexedrine	Swollen patches, itchy skin
Equanil	Rash, welts, dermatitis
Librium	Pimples
Miltown	Welts, flaking skin, itching
Nembutal	Skin rash
Phenobarbital	Rash, itchy skin, swollen eyelids
Placidyl	Itchy skin, swollen patches

Quaalude	Pimples, welts
Talwin	Rash, facial swelling, skin peeling
Tetracycline	Taken during pregnancy and in infancy may cause permanent discoloration of child's teeth
Thorazine	Peeling skin, jaundice, welts, swelling
Tofranil	Rash, itchy skin, jaundice
Tuinal	Can aggravate existing skin condition
Valium	Jaundice, rash, swollen patches

265. Any Questions About Chapter XIX?

What do you think of jojoba oil as a beauty aid?

Personally, I think it's one of the best. It's available in a variety of forms—an oil, a cream, a soap, a shampoo—and it works wonders naturally!

For example: As a moisturizer, use a few drops under your makeup. Massage gently into your skin, particularly around the eyes where lines occur. (Be careful to avoid direct contact with the eyes and if any irritation results, discontinue use.) At night, use the oil to soften your skin as you sleep. Just apply a light layer over your face and neck—after they've had a good cleansing, of course.

The oil can also be used to soften skin after showers (all you need is a few drops) and as a luxuriant bath oil (again, just a few drops). For dry, chapped, or recently shaved skin, it should be applied directly.

After shampooing your hair, try rubbing a few drops of the oil into your hair and scalp (don't rinse). Daily use will help even the dryest hair return to its natural luster.

My nails just won't grow. I've tried all sorts of vitamins, but they don't work. Where do I go from here?

It's possible that you might have a thyroid problem, so you might want to check with a nutritionally oriented physician (see section 278).

In the meanwhile, you could try silica, an organic herb that's also known as horsetail and *Equisetum arvense*, which is changed by the body into readily available calcium—which nourishes nails, skin, hair, bones, and the body's connective tissue.

XX

Staying Young, Energetic, and Sexy

266. Retarding the Aging Process

Aging is caused by the degeneration of cells. Our bodies are made up of millions of these cells, each with a life of somewhere around two years or less. But before a cell dies, it reproduces itself. Why, then, you might wonder, shouldn't we look the same now as we did ten years ago? The reason for this is that with each successive reproduction, the cell goes through some alteration—basically, deterioration. So as our cells change, deteriorate, we grow old.

> You can look and feel six
> to twelve years younger.

Dr. Benjamin S. Frank, author of *Nucleic Acid Therapy in Aging and Degenerative Disease*, has found that deteriorating cells can be rejuvenated if provided with substances that directly nourish them—substances such as nucleic acids.

DNA (deoxyribonucleic acid) and RNA (ribonucleic

acid) are our nucleic acids. DNA is essentially a chemical boilerplate for new cells. It sends out RNA molecules like a team of well-trained workers to form them. When DNA stops giving the orders to RNA, new cell construction ceases—as does life. But by helping the body stay well supplied with nucleic acids, Dr. Frank has found that you can look and feel six to twelve years younger than you actually are.

According to Dr. Frank, we need 1 to 1.5 g. of nucleic acid daily. Though the body can produce its own nucleic acids, he feels they are broken down too quickly into less useful compounds and should be supplied from external sources if the aging process is to be retarded, even reversed.

Foods rich in nucleic acids are wheat germ, bran, spinach, asparagus, mushrooms, fish (especially sardines, salmon, and anchovies), chicken liver, oatmeal, and onions. He recommends a diet where seafood is eaten seven times a week, along with two glasses of skimmed milk, a glass of fruit or vegetable juice, and four glasses of water daily.

After only two months of RNA-DNA supplementation and diet, Dr. Frank found that his patients had more energy and that there was a substantial diminution of lines and wrinkles, with healthier, rosier, and younger-looking skin in evidence.

One of the most recent arrivals in the battle to combat aging is SOD (superoxide dismutase). This enzyme fortifies the body against the ravages of free radicals, destructive molecules that speed the aging process by destroying healthy cells as well as attacking collagen (''cement'' that holds cells together).

As we age, our bodies produce less SOD, so supplementation—along with a natural diet that restricts free radical formation—can help increase our energetic and productive years. It's important to note, though, that SOD can become inactive very quickly if essential minerals, such as zinc, copper, and manganese, are not supplied.

DHEA (dehydroepiandrosterone), a natural hormone that is produced by the adrenal glands, is now also being used in antiaging regimens, since one of its properties is that it can "de-excite" the body's processes and thereby slow down the production of fats, hormones, and acids that contribute to aging.

267. Basic Keep Yourself Young Program

Along with proper diet, a good supplement regimen is important to the success of looking, feeling, and keeping yourself young.

High-potency multiple vitamin with chelated minerals (time release preferred) A.M. and P.M.

Vitamin C, 1,000 mg. with bioflavonoids A.M. and P.M.

Vitamin E (dry form), 400 IU with antioxidants A.M. and P.M.

RNA-DNA, 100-mg. tablets, 1 daily for one month, then 2 daily for the next month, then 3 daily thereafter, 6 days a week

Stress B complex, A.M. and P.M.

SOD, 125 mcg., 1 daily for one month, then 2 daily for the next month, then 3 daily thereafter, 6 days a week

DHEA, 1 daily, an hour before meals for one month; 2 daily, an hour before meals, second month; 3 daily, an hour before meals, thereafter—6 days a week

268. High-Pep Energy Regimen

Whether you want to feel good or just look good, exercise, diet, and the right supplements are the tickets to high energy.

If you're not into jogging, can't afford the sneakers, don't play tennis, find yourself reluctant to swim in twenty-below weather, and hate calisthenics, I have the perfect exercise for you—jumping rope.

A jump rope is inexpensive, convenient (you can take it everywhere), and lots of fun to use. And it works! In terms of calories burned, jumping rope can outdo bicycling, tennis, and swimming. An average person of about 150 pounds uses up 720 calories an hour jumping rope (120 to 140 turns per minute). When you realize that an hour of tennis uses up only 420 calories, you have a better idea of just how good jumping rope can be for you.

For keeping energy high, remember to eat a combination of two protein foods (or a protein drink) at each meal; drink at least six glasses of water daily (a half hour before or after meals); avoid refined sugar, flour, tobacco, alcohol, tea, coffee, soft drinks, processed and fried foods.

A good pep-up protein drink:

1 tbsp. protein powder
1 tbsp. lecithin granules
2 tbsp. acidophilus liquid
1 tbsp. nutritional yeast
1 tbsp. safflower oil (optional)

Blend with milk, water, or juice in blender for 1 minute. (Add fresh fruit if desired.)

269. High-Pep Supplements

With breakfast:

High-potency multiple vitamin with chelated minerals
(time release preferred)
Vitamin E (dry form), 400 IU
High-potency multiple chelated mineral
Acidophilus, 3 capsules or 2 tbsp. liquid
Lecithin granules, 1 tbsp. or 3 1,200 mg. capsules
3 calcium and magnesium tablets

With lunch:

Acidophilus, 3 capsules or 2 tbsp. liquid
Lecithin granules, 1 tbsp. or 3 1,200 mg. capsules
Optional: vitamin B_{12}, liver tablets, digestive enzymes

With dinner:

Vitamin E (dry form), 400 IU
Acidophilus, 3 capsules or 2 tbsp. liquid
Lecithin granules, 1 tbsp. or 3 1,200 mg. capsules
Optional: digestive enzymes

270. Vitamins and Sex

The important thing to remember is that if you're not
feeling up to par, your sex drive is going to suffer along
with the rest of you.

There have been many claims for vitamin E in relation to sex. Studies have indeed shown that it increases
the fertility in males and females and helps restore male
potency. That it strongly influences the sex drive in men

and women has yet to be proven, though I have met many vitamin-E takers who are happily convinced that it does.

> The largest percentage of zinc
> in a man's body is found in
> the prostate.

Another noteworthy sex nutrient is zinc. The largest percentage of zinc in a man's body is found in the prostate, and a lack of the mineral can produce testicular atrophy and prostate trouble.

Remember, vitamins that keep up your energy levels (see sections 268, 269) will also do a lot for your sexual performance.

271. Food and Supplements for Better Sex

Oysters (yes, they're high in zinc), shellfish of all kinds, brewer's yeast, wheat bran, wheat germ, whole grains, and pumpkin seeds. Incorporating these foods in a program that includes a high-protein and basically low-carbohydrate diet, exercise, and supplements is as good as an aphrodisiac for lovers.

Supplements
MVP (see section 128)
Vitamin B complex, 50 mg., 1–3 times daily
Vitamin E, 400 IU, 1–3 times daily
Zinc, 50 mg. (chelated), 1–3 times daily
Ginseng, 500 mg., 3 times daily 1 hour before meals

272. Any Questions About Chapter XX?

I understand that octacosanol can improve a male's sexual performance enormously. What do you feel about this?

I feel that a lot is still going to depend on the male involved. It is true, though, that octacosanol (which is a natural food substance present in very small amounts in many vegetable oils, the leaves of alfalfa and wheat, wheat germ, and other foods) has an energy-releasing function, increasing strength and stamina, and in laboratory experiments it seems to improve reproductive disturbances.

If you try it, don't be impatient, it often takes 4 to 6 weeks for beneficial effects from octacosanol to be noticed.

Always keep in mind, too, that an energizing diet of raw or lightly cooked foods, rich in B vitamins and amino acids, will contribute to a good sex life.

XXI

Pets Need Good Nutrition, Too

273. Vitamins for Your Dog

Dogs need vitamins as much as people do. Their requirements, of course, are not the same as ours, but they, too, need all the nutrients. (If you want to know exactly what they need for basic nutrition, write for the National Research Council's *Nutrient Requirements for Dogs,* National Academy of Sciences, Washington, DC.)

An adult dog needs 4.4 g. protein daily, along with 1.3 g. fat, 0.4 g. linoleic or arachidonic acid, and 15.4 g. carbohydrate. Puppies need twice that amount.

Proteins are essential for a dog's growth and body repair. Those with a high biological value, such as eggs, muscle meat, fish meat, soybeans, milk, and yeast, are the best. If you want to give your dog eggs, be sure that they're cooked. Raw egg white contains avidin, which prevents biotin from being absorbed. Milk, though good for dogs, often causes diarrhea, so yogurt and cottage cheese are recommended.

Carbohydrates are used by dogs for energy, but it is suggested that no more than 50 to 60 percent of their food include them.

Fats, the most concentrated energy source, supply the

essential fatty acid for healthy skin and hair. A deficiency can retard puppies' growth and lead to coarse hair and flaking skin. One teaspoon of safflower or corn oil added to the dog's dry food can help.

Imbalanced supplements can
harm your dog.

Calcium and phosphorus, in a ratio of 1.2 to 1, should be included in the dog's diet. If the ratio is incorrect, abnormal mineralization can occur in the bones of growing puppies as well as adult dogs. There must also be sufficient vitamin D for proper absorption of these two minerals. Because the balance is so important, *be certain that the vitamin supplements you give are balanced.* Too much bonemeal or cod liver oil can result in problems as severe as those you're trying to combat.

Cod liver oil is not advised as a routine supplement; it can lead to vitamin-D overload.

All-meat diets are not good for your pet because the calcium-phosphorus ratio is wrong and there are inadequate amounts of vitamins A, D, and E.

Stop fleas with brewer's
yeast.

Brewer's yeast, mixed in with your dog's food, will help prevent fleas. (It works for cats, too.) Fleas despise the odor it gives off after your dog ingests it.

Do not give your dog supplemental vitamins A, D, or niacin. They can have an adverse effect on the animal. (See section 277 for "Cautions.")

274. Arthritis and Dysplasia Regimen for Dogs

Dogs, unlike humans, manufacture their own vitamin C, but recent reseach has shown that supplemental C can be effective in the treatment of arthritis and dysplasia. I recommend, though, that you consult your vet before starting any vitamin program. Ask him or her about this regimen:

Vitamin C, 300 mg.
4–5 alfalfa tablets
Vitamin E, 100 IU
Mix with food daily

275. Vitamins for Your Cat

Cats need vitamins, just as people and dogs do, but nutritional requirements for them have not been as well established. (For the most recent available information, you can write for the National Research Council's *Nutrient Requirements of Laboratory Animals*, National Academy of Sciences, Washington, DC.)

Cow's milk is insufficient
for a growing kitten.

Protein requirements for cats are high, considerably higher than those of dogs or people. And kittens need one-third more protein than adult cats. Muscle meats, organ meat, poultry, fish, cheese, eggs, and milk are all good sources. (Eggs should be cooked or, if given raw, only the yolk should be used.) If you are giving a kitten milk, use a dry powdered milk at double the concentration given a human baby; cow's milk isn't nutritious enough for an infant cat.

Carbohydrates are not actually required in a cat's diet, but they are used as energy. If there are adequate levels of fats and protein, 33 percent of the diet can be made up of carbohydrates.

Give your cat the fats
you shouldn't eat.

Fats are a cat's most concentrated source of energy. Unlike people, cats can have diets of up to 64 percent fat and show no signs of vascular problems. Only because fats are more costly than carbohydrates do most cat foods have low percentages. In fact, you can give your cat the fats you need to cut down on—butter, animal fat, vegetable. Where cats are concerned, polyunsaturates are not the good guys. Too much polyunsaturated fatty acid is antagonistic to vitamin E, and fat deposits in the cat's body can be seriously affected.

Although levels of all the essential vitamins haven't been established for cats, the importance of certain vitamins in a cat's diet should be noted. For example, cats are dependent on their diet for fully formed vitamin A (their requirement is much higher than that of dogs because unlike dogs they cannot manufacture vitamin A in the body from carotene). On the other hand, too much vitamin A can result in bone deformities. Liver as a supplement (not a total diet) is recommended, as is a *balanced* vitamin-mineral preparation. Fish, butter, milk, and cheese are also high in vitamin A.

The B vitamins are also important for a cat's nerve stability, outer coat, and inner tissues. B_6 (pyridoxine) helps prevent urinary calculi, a serious problem for altered male cats. (A diet low in ash is recommended.)

In general, cats require twice the amount of B vitamins needed by dogs, and feeding dog food to a cat for an extended period of time can result in a B-complex deficiency. It should also be noted that B_1 (thiamine) can be destroyed by an antagonist in raw fish. (For foods high in B vitamins, see sections 27, 28, and 29.)

> All-fish diets are not
> healthy for cats.

Vitamin-E deficiency can occur from feeding excessive amounts of red meat tuna (it can also occur because of any all-fish diet). Lack of appetite, fever, pain, and a reluctance to move are characteristic symptoms of pansteatitis, which results from vitamin-E deficiency. If this occurs, see your vet, don't feed tuna unless it is supplemented with vitamin E, and don't use fish oils as supplements.

The calcium-phosphorus ratio in a cat's diet should be about one to one, with adequate amounts of vitamin D. Since manufacturers of canned cat foods usually add irradiated yeast, a source of vitamin D, supplements of D are unnecessary— and can be dangerous. (See section 277 for "Cautions.")

A multiple vitamin with iron—prepared especially for cats—is often given for feline anemia. The disease is rare in cats on a balanced diet that includes cooked and raw muscle meat, organ meats, cooked or canned chicken, and fish, vitamin-rich cereals, and vegetables.

Keep in mind that pregnant or lactating cats, who often eat 10 to 15 ounces of food a day, have double or triple the vitamin requirements of an average five- to seven-pound cat.

276. Any Questions About Chapter XXI?

If selenium is an important antioxidant for humans, shouldn't it be given to dogs who live in cities, too?

I would not recommend selenium supplementation for dogs or cats unless such supplementation is prescribed by a vet and carefully monitored. Casual supplementation can be hazardous, particularly if your pet is old or sick.

XXII

Vitamin "Yeses" and "Nos" You Should Know

277. Cautions

Though we all know that vitamins are good for us, there are times, situations, and metabolic conditions where caution and special adjustments are advised. I recommend you look over the following list carefully for your own well-being and in order to get the most from your vitamins.

• Chronic hypervitaminosis A can occur in patients receiving megadoses as treatment for dermatological conditions.

• A deficiency of vitamin A can lead to loss of vitamin C.

• An oversupply of vitamin B_1 (thiamine) can affect thyroid and insulin production and might cause B_6 deficiency, as well as loss of other B vitamins.

• Prolonged ingestion of any B vitamin can result in significant depletion of the others.

• Pregnant women should check with their doctors before taking sustained doses of over 50 mg. of vitamin B_6 (pyridoxine).

• B_6 should not be taken by anyone under L-dopa treatment for Parkinson's disease.

• Large doses of vitamin B_2 (riboflavin), especially if taken without antioxidant supplements, may cause a sensitivity to sunlight.

• Because vitamin D promotes absorption of calcium, a large excess of stored vitamin D can cause too much calcium in the blood (hypercalcemia).

• Don't eat raw egg whites. They deactivate the body's biotin.

• It is possible that large amounts of vitamin C might reverse the anticoagulant activity of the blood thinner warfarin, commonly prescribed as the drug Coumadin.

• Diabetes and heart patients should check with their doctors, because vitamin C might necessitate a lower dosage of pills.

• Megadoses of vitamin C wash out B_{12} and folic acid, so be sure you are taking at least the daily requirement of both.

• Excessive doses of choline, taken over a long period of time, may produce a deficiency of vitamin B_6.

• If you have a heart disorder, check with your physician for the proper vitamin-D dosage to take.

• Vitamin E should be used cautiously by anyone with an overactive thyroid, diabetes, high blood pressure, or rheumatic heart disease. (If you have any of these conditions, start at a very low dosage and build up gradually by 100 IU daily each month to between 400 and 800 IU.)

• Rheumatic heart fever sufferers should know that they have an imbalance between the two sides of their hearts and large vitamin-E doses can increase the imbalance and worsen the condition. (Before using supplements, consult your physician.)

• Vitamin E can elevate blood pressure in hypertensives, but if supplementation is started with a low dosage and increased slowly, the end result will be an eventual lowering of the pressure through the vitamin's diuretic properties.

• Diabetics have been able to reduce their insulin levels with E. Check with your physician.

• Decreases in vitamin E should be gradual, too.

• An excessive intake of folic acid can mask symptoms of pernicious anemia.

• High doses of folic acid for extended periods of time are not recommended for anyone with a medical history of convulsive disorders or hormone-related cancer.

• Folic acid and PABA might inhibit the effectiveness of sulfonamides, such as Gantrisin.

• Megadoses of vitamin K can build up and cause a red cell breakdown and anemia.

• Patients on the blood thinner Dicumarol should be aware that synthetic K could counteract the effectiveness of the drug. Conversely, the drug inhibits the absorption of natural vitamin K.

• Sweats and flushes can occur from too much vitamin K.

• Niacin should be used cautiously by anyone with severe diabetes, glaucoma, peptic ulcers, or with impaired liver function.

• Do not give niacin to your dog or cat; it causes flushing and sweating and greatly discomforts the animal. Do not supplement a pet's diet with vitamins A or D unless your vet specifically advises it.

• Excessive amounts of PABA (para-aminobenzoic acid) in certain individuals can have a negative effect on the liver, kidneys, and heart.

• Iron should not be taken by anyone with sickle-cell anemia, hemochromatosis, or thalassemia.

• If your iron supplement is ferrous sulfate, you're losing vitamin E.

• Large quantities of caffeine can inhibit iron absorption.

• Anyone with kidney malfunction should not take more than 3,000 mg. of magnesium on a daily basis.

• Too much manganese will reduce utilization of the body's iron.

• High doses of manganese can cause motor difficulties and weakness in certain individuals.

• Diet high in fat increase phosphorus absorption and lower your calcium levels.

• If you take cortisone and aldosterone drugs, such as Aldactone and prednisone, you lose potassium and retain sodium. Check with your physician for proper supplements.

• Excessive perspiration can cause a depletion of sodium.

• Too much sodium can cause a potassium loss.

• Excessive zinc intakes can result in iron and copper losses.

• If you add zinc to your diet, be sure you're getting enough vitamin A.

• Anyone suffering from Wilson's disease is susceptible to copper toxicity.

• Too much cobalt may cause an unwanted enlargement of the thyroid gland.

• Anyone taking thyroid medication should be aware that kelp also affects that gland. If you have been using both, a consultation with your doctor and retesting are advised. You might need *less* prescription medicine than you think.

• Large amounts of raw cabbage can cause an iodine

deficiency and throw off thyroid production in individuals with existing low-iodine intakes.

• Milk that contains synthetic vitamin D can deplete the body of magnesium.

• Heavy coffee and tea drinkers—cola drinkers, too—should be aware that large caffeine ingestion creates an inositol shortage.

• Inform your doctor if you're taking large amounts of vitamin C. C can change results of lab tests for sugar in the blood and urine and give false negative results in tests for blood in stool specimens.

• Don't engage in strenuous physical activity within four hours after taking vitamin A if you want optimum absorption.

• Copper has a tendency to accumulate in the blood and deplete the brain's zinc supplies.

• Tryptophan should not be taken with protein; use juice or water to swallow tablets, not milk.

• RNA-DNA supplements increase serum uric acid levels and should *not* be taken by anyone with gout.

• Tyrosine and phenylalanine may increase blood pressure and should *not* be taken with MAO inhibitors or other antidepressant drugs. These amino acids are also contraindicated for anyone with pigmented malignant melanomas.

• PABA is contraindicated with *methotrexate* (Mexate), a cancer-fighting drug.

• Folacin (folic acid) decreases the anticonvulsant action of *phenytoin* (Dilantin).

• Antibiotics are reduced in their effectiveness when taken with supplements. (Take supplements at least an hour before or two hours after prescription antibiotics.)

• Calcium can interfere with the effectiveness of tetracycline.
• High doses of vitamin D or calcium ascorbate are contraindicated if you are taking the heart medication *digoxin* (Lanoxin).
• Broad spectrum antibiotics should not be taken with high doses of vitamin A.
• Vitamin A should not be taken in conjunction with the acne drug Accutane (*isotretinoin*).
• Choline is not recommended during the depressive phase of manic-depressive conditions, since it can deepen this particular sort of depression.
• Papaya, as well as raw pineapple, is not recommended for anyone with an ulcer.

XXIII

Locating a Nutritionally Oriented Doctor

278. How to Go About It

For a list of nutritionally oriented practitioners in your area, write to the following organizations. Be sure to enclose a stamped, self-addressed envelope.

International College of Applied Nutrition
Box 386
La Habra, California 90631

International Academy of Preventative Medicine
10950 Grandview, Suite 469
Overland Park, Kansas 66210

International Academy of Metabiology, Inc.
P.O. Box 15157
Las Cruces, New Mexico 88001

Prevention Magazine Reader's Service
Emmaus, Pennsylvania 18049

Orthomolecular Medical Society
6151 West Century Boulevard
Suite 1114
Los Angeles, California 90045

Afterword

As more and more people have become aware of the importance of vitamins in their daily lives, the need for clear, uncomplicated information has become evident. And with recent research showing that the right vitamins at the right time are much more important to us than anyone ever realized, the need has become a necessity. It is my hope that this newly revised book has fulfilled that need, that it has debunked the myths surrounding food and nutrition and erased any uncertainties about the nature, function, and safety of vitamins.

Whether you have read the book cover to cover or simply thumbed through to personally relevant points, I believe you'll find its reference value will increase as new life situations arise. My intention was to provide an omnibus guide that could answer not only your present vitamin questions, but future ones as well. As time goes by, the sections on staying young, energetic, and sexy, and retarding the aging process will bear rereading, as will those offering regimens for whatever your new particular circumstances happens to be. In other words, the information I have set down is meant to be perused and is intended not just for today, but for many, many happy and healthy tomorrows.

Earl L. Mindell, R.Ph. Ph.d.

Beverly Hills, California
August 30, 1984

Glossary

Absorption: the process by which nutrients are passed into the bloodstream.

Acetate: a derivative of acetic acid.

Acetic acid: used as a synthetic flavoring agent, one of the first food additives (vinegar is approximately 4 to 6 percent acetic acid); it is found naturally in cheese, coffee, grapes, peaches, raspberries, and strawberries; Generally Recognized As Safe (GRAS) when used only in packaging.

Acetone: a colorless solvent for fat, oils, and waxes, which is obtained by fermentation (inhalation can irritate lungs, and large amounts have a narcotic effect).

Acid: a water-soluble substance with a sour taste.

Adrenals: the glands, located above each kidney, that manufacture adrenaline.

Alkali: an acid-neutralizing substance (sodium bicarbonate is an alkali used for excess acidity in foods).

Allergen: a substance that causes an allergy.

Alzheimer's disease: a progressively degenerative disease, involved with loss of memory, which new research indicates might be helped with extra choline.

Amino acid chelates: chelated minerals that have been produced by many of the same processes nature uses to chelate minerals in the body; in the digestive tract, nature surrounds the elemental minerals with amino acid, permitting them to be absorbed into the bloodstream.

Amino acids: the organic compounds from which proteins are constructed; there are twenty-two known amino acids, but only nine are indispensable nutrients for man—histidine, isoleucine, leucine, lysine, total S-containing amino acids, total aromatic amino acids, threonine, tryptophan, and valine.

Anorexia: loss of appetite.

Antibiotic: any of various substances that are effective in inhibiting or destroying bacteria.

Anticoagulant: something that delays or prevents blood clotting.

Antigen: any substance not normally present in the body that stimulates the body to produce antibodies.

Antihistamine: a drug used to reduce effects associated with histamine production in allergies and colds.

Antioxidant: a substance that can protect another substance from oxidation; added to foods to keep oxygen from changing the food's color.

Antitoxin: an antibody formed in response to, and capable of neutralizing, a poison of biologic origin.

Assimilation: the process whereby nutrients are used by the body and changed into living tissue.

Ataxia: loss of coordinated movement caused by disease of nervous system.

ATP: a molecule called adenozine triphosphate, the fuel of life, a nucleotide—building block of nucleic acid—that produces biological energy with B_1, B_2, B_3, and pantothenic acid.

Avidin: a protein in egg white capable of inactivating biotin.

Bariatrician: a weight-control doctor.

B cells: white blood cells, made in the bone marrow, which produce antibodies upon instructions from T cells, white blood cells manufactured in the thymus.

BHA: butylated hydroxyanisole; a preservative and antioxidant used in many products; insoluble in water; can be toxic to the kidneys.

BHT: butylated hydroxytoluene; a solid, white crystalline antioxidant used to retard spoilage of many foods; can be more toxic to the kidney than its nearly identical chemical cousin BHA.

Bioflavonoids: usually from orange and lemon rinds, these citrus-flavored compounds needed to maintain healthy blood-vessel walls are widely available in plants, citrus fruits, and rose hips; known as vitamin P complex.

Calciferol: a colorless, odorless crystalline material, insoluble in water; soluble in fats; a synthetic form of vitamin D made by irradiating ergosterol with ultraviolet light.

Calcium gluconate: an organic form of calcium.

Capillary: a minute blood vessel, one of many that connect the arteries and veins.

Carcinogen: a cancer-causing substance.

Carotene: an orange-yellow pigment occurring in many plants and capable of being converted into vitamin A in the body.

Casein: the protein in milk that has become the standard by which protein quality is measured.

Catabolism: the metabolic change of nutrients or complex substances into simpler compounds, accompanied by a release of energy.

Catalyst: a substance that modifies, especially increases, the rate of chemical reaction without being consumed or changed in the process.

Chelation: a process by which mineral substances are changed into easily digestible form.

Chronic: a long duration; continuing; constant.

CNS: central nervous system.

Coenzyme: the major portion, though nonprotein, of an enzyme; usually a B vitamin.

Collagen: the primary organic constituent of bone, cartilage, and connective tissue (becomes gelatin through boiling).

Congenital: condition existing at birth, not hereditary.

Dehydration: a condition resulting from an excessive loss of water from the body.

Dermatitis: an inflammation of the skin; a rash.

Desiccated: dried; preserved by removing moisture.

Dicalcium phosphate: a filler used in pills, which is derived from purified mineral rocks and is an excellent source of calcium and phosphorus.

Diluents: fillers; inert material added to tablets to increase their bulk in order to make them a practical size for compression.

Diuretic: tending to increase the flow of urine from the body.

DNA: deoxyribonucleic acid; the nucleic acid in chromosomes that is part of the chemical basis for hereditary characteristics.

Endogenous: being produced from within the body.

Enteric coated: a tablet coated so that it dissolves in the intestine, not in the stomach (which is acid).

Enuresis: bed-wetting.

Enzyme: a protein substance found in living cells that brings about chemical changes; necessary for digestion of food.

Excipient: any inert substance used as a dilutant or vehicle for a drug.

Exogenous: being derived or developed from external causes.

FDA: Food and Drug Administration.

Fibrin: an insoluble protein that forms the necessary fibrous network in the coagulation of blood.

Free radicals: highly reactive chemical fragments that can produce an irritation of artery walls, start the arteriosclerotic process if vitamin E is not present; generally harmful.

Fructose: a natural sugar occurring in fruits and honey; called fruit sugar; often used as a preservative for foodstuffs and an intravenous nutrient.

Galactosemia: a hereditary disorder in which milk becomes toxic as food.

Glucose: blood sugar; a product of the body's assimilation of carbohydrates and a major source of energy.

Glutamic acid: an amino acid present in all complete proteins; usually manufactured from vegetable protein; used as a salt substitute and a flavor-intensifying agent.

Glutamine: an amino acid that constitutes, with glucose, the major nourishment used by the nervous system.

Gluten: a mixture of two proteins—gliadin and glutenin—present in wheat, rye, oats, and barley.

Glycogen: the body's chief storage carbohydrate, primarily in the liver.

GRAS: Generally Recognized As Safe; a list established by Congress to cover substances added to food.

Hesperidin: part of the C complex.

Holistic treatment: treatment of the whole person.

Homeostasis: the body's physiological equilibrium.

Hormone: a substance formed in endocrine organs and transported by body fluids to activate other specifically receptive organs.

Humectant: a substance that is used to preserve the moisture content of materials.

Hydrochloric acid: a normally acidic part of the body's gastric juice.

Hydrolyzed: put into water-soluble form.

Hydrolyzed protein chelate: water soluble and chelated for easy assimilation.

Hypervitaminosis: a condition caused by an excessive ingestion of vitamins.

Hypoglycemia: a condition caused by abnormally low blood sugar.

Hypovitaminosis: a deficiency disease owing to an absence of vitamins in the diet.

Ichthyosis: a condition characterized by a scaliness on the outer layer of skin.

Idiopathic: a condition whose causes are not yet known.

Immune: protected against disease.

Insulin: the hormone, secreted by the pancreas, concerned with the metabolism of sugar in the body.

IU: international units.

Lactating: producing milk.

Laxative: a substance that stimulates evacuation of the bowels.

Linoleic acid: one of the polyunsaturated fats, a constituent of lecithin; known as vitamin F; indispensable for life and must be obtained from foods.

Lipid: a fat or fatty substance.

Lipofuscin: age pigment in cells.

Lipotropic: preventing abnormal or excessive accumulation of fat in the liver.

Megavitamin therapy: treatment of illness with massive amounts of vitamins.

Metabolize: to undergo change by physical and chemical processes.

Mucopolysaccharide: thick gelatinous material that is found many places in the body; it glues cells together and lubricates joints.

Nitrites: used as fixatives in cured meats; can combine with natural stomach and food chemicals to cause dangerous cancer-causing agents called nitrosamines.

Orthomolecular: the right molecule used for the right treatment; doctors who practice preventive medicine and use vitamin therapies are known as orthomolecular physicians.

OSHA: Occupational Safety and Health Administration.

Oxalates: organic chemicals found in certain foods, especially spinach, which can combine with calcium to form calcium oxalate, an insoluble chemical the body cannot use.

PABA: para-aminobenzoic acid; a member of the B complex.

Palmitate: water-solubilized vitamin A.

PKU (phenylketonuria): a hereditary disease caused by the lack of an enzyme needed to convert an essential amino acid (phenylalanine) into a form usable by the body; can cause mental retardation unless detected early.

Polyunsaturated fats: highly nonsaturated fats from vegetable sources; tend to lower blood cholesterol.

Predigested protein: protein that has been processed for fast assimilation and can go directly to the bloodstream.

Provitamin: a vitamin precursor; a chemical substance necessary to produce a vitamin.

PUFA: polyunsaturated fatty acid.

RDA: Recommended Dietary Allowances as established by the Food and Nutrition Board, National Academy of Sciences, National Research Council.

RNA: the abbreviation used for ribonucleic acid.

Rose hips: a rich source of vitamin C; the nodule underneath the bud of a rose called a hip, in which the plant produces the vitamin C we extract.

Rutin: a substance extracted from buckwheat; part of the C complex.

Saturated fatty acids: usually solid at room temperature; higher proportions found in foods from animal sources; tend to raise blood cholesterol levels.

Sequestrant: a substance that absorbs ions and prevents changes that would affect flavor, texture, and color of food; used for water softening.

Syncope: brief loss of consciousness; fainting.

Synergistic: the action of two or more substances to produce an effect that neither alone could accomplish.

Synthetic: produced artificially.

Systemic: capable of spreading through the entire body.

T cells: white blood cells, manufactured in the thymus, which protect the body from bacteria, viruses, and cancer-causing agents, while controlling the production of B cells, which produce antibodies, and unwanted production of potentially harmful T cells.

Teratological: monstrous or abnormal formations in animals or plants.

Tocopherols: the group of compounds (alpha, beta, delta, episilon, eta, gamma, and zeta) that make vitamin E; obtained through vacuum distillation of edible vegetable oils.

Toxicity: the quality or condition of being poisonous, harmful, or destructive.

Toxin: an organic poison produced in living or dead organisms.

Triglycerides: fatty substances in the blood.

Unsaturated fatty acids: most often liquid at room temperature; primarily found in vegetable fats.

USAN: United States Adopted Names Council; cosponsored by the American Pharmaceutical Association (APhA), the American Medical Association (AMA), and the United States Pharmacopeia (USP) for the specific purpose of coining suitable, acceptable, nonproprietary names in the drug field.

USRDA: United States Recommended Daily Allowances.

Xerosis: a condition of dryness.

Zein: protein from corn.

Zyme: a fermenting substance.

Bibliography and
Recommended Reading

I owe a great debt of thanks to the many scientists, doctors, nutritionists, professors, and researchers whose painstaking and all too often unrewarding work in the field of vitamins and nutrition has made this book possible.

The following list is given to show my sincere appreciation and make known the foundation upon which I have built my knowledge. Many of the books are highly technical and confusing for the layman, meant as they are for professionals in the field. But others, which I have marked with an asterisk, I heartily commend to you for further reading and a healthier future.

*Abrahamson, E. M., and Pezet, A. W. *Body, Mind and Sugar*. New York: Avon Books, 1977.

*Adams, Ruth. *The Complete Home Guide to All the Vitamins*. New York: Larchmont Books, 1972.

*Adams, Ruth, and Murray, Frank. *Minerals: Kill or Cure*. New York: Larchmont Books, 1976.

*Aguilar, Nona. *Totally Natural Beauty*. New York: Rawson Associates Publishers, 1977.

*Airola, Paavo. *Are You Confused?* Phoenix, AZ: Health Plus, 1972.

*————. *How to Get Well*. Phoenix, AZ; Health Plus, 1975.

*————. *Hypoglycemia, a Better Approach*. Phoenix, AZ: Health Plus, 1977.

Amberson, Rosanne. *Raising Your Cat*. New York: Bonanza Books, 1969.

*Atkins, Robert C. *Dr. Atkins' Diet Revolution*. New York: David McKay, 1972.

*Bailey, Hubert. *Vitamin E. Your Key to a Healthy Heart*. New York: ARC Books, 1964, 1966.

Bieri, John G. "Fat-soluble vitamins in the eighth revision of the Recommended Dietary Allowances." *Journal of the American Dietetic Association* 64 (February 1974).

Blood: The River of Life. American National Red Cross, 1976.

*Borsaak, Henry. *Vitamins: What They Are and How They Can Benefit You*. New York: Pyramid Books, 1971.

"Bread: You Can't Judge a Loaf by Its Color." *Consumer Reports* 41 (May 1976).

*Bricklin, Mark. *Practical Encyclopedia of Natural Healing*. Emmaus, PA: Rodale Press, 1976.

Brody, Jane E. "Cancer-blocking Agents Found in Foods." *New York Times*, 6 March 1979.

*————. *The New York Times Guide to Personal Health*. New York: Times Books, 1982.

*Burack, Richard, with Fox, Fred J. *New Handbook of Prescription Drugs*. New York: Pantheon Books, 1967.

Burton, Benjamin. *Human Nutrition*. 3rd ed. New York: McGraw-Hill, 1976.

"Buying Beef." *Consumer Reports* 39 (September 1974).

*Carr, William H. A. *The Basic Book of the Cat*. New York: Gramercy Publishing Co., 1963.

*Chapman, Esther. *How to Use the 12 Tissue Salts*. New York: Pyramid Books, 1977.

*Clark, Linda. *The Best of Linda Clark*. New Canaan, CT: Keats Publishing Co., 1976.

*————. *Know Your Nutrition*. New Canaan, CT: Keats Publishing Co., 1973.

*————. *Secrets of Health and Beauty*. New York: Jove Publication, 1977.

*Consumer Reports, Editors of. *The Medicine Show*. Mount Vernon, NY: Consumers Union, 1981.

Cooper, Barber, Mitchell, Rynberge, Green. *Nutrition in Health and Disease*. New York: Lippincott, 1963.

Cumulative Index for Journal of Applied Nutrition. La Habra, CA: International College of Applied Nutrition, 1947–76, 1976.

*Davis, Adelle. *Let's Eat Right to Keep Fit*. New York: Harcourt, Brace and World, 1954.

*————. *Let's Get Well*. New York: Harcourt, Brace and World, 1965.

*————. *Let's Have Healthy Children*. 2nd ed. New York: Harcourt, Brace and World, 1959.

*Dufty, William. *Sugar Blues*. Pennsylvania: Chilton Book Co., 1975.

*Ebon, Martin. *Which Vitamins Do You Need?* New York: Bantam Books, 1974.

Flynn, Margaret A. "The Cholesterol Controversy." *Journal of the American Pharmacy* NS18 (May 1978).

"Food Facts Talk Back." *Journal of the American Dietetic Association*, 1977.

*Frank, Benjamin S. *No-Aging Diet*. New York: Dial, 1976.

*Fredericks, Carlton. *Eating Right for You*. New York: Grosset and Dunlap, 1972.

*———. *Look Younger/Feel Healthier*. New York: Grosset and Dunlap, 1977.

*———. *Psycho Nutrients*. New York: Grosset and Dunlap, 1975.

*Gomez, Joan, and Gerch, Marvin J. *Dictionary of Symptoms*. New York: Stein and Day, 1963.

Goodhart, Robert S., and Shills, Maurice E. *Modern Nutrition in Health and Disease*. 5th ed. Philadelphia: Lea and Febiger, 1973.

*Graedon, Joe. *The People's Pharmcy*. New York: St. Martin's Press, 1976.

Guidelines for the Eradication of Iron Deficiency Anemia. New York: International Nutritional Anemia Consultative Group (INACG), 1976.

Guidelines for the Eradication of Vitamin-A Deficiency and Xerophthalmia. International Vitamin-A Consultative Group (IVACG).

Harper, Alfred E. "Recommended Dietary Allowances: Are They What We Think They Are?" *Journal of the American Dietetic Association* 64 (February 1974).

Holvey, David, ed. *The Merck Manual*. 12th ed. Rahway, NJ: Merck and Co., 1972.

Howe, Phyllis S. *Basic Nutrition in Health and Disease*. 6th ed. Philadelphia: W. B. Saunders Co., 1976.

"How Nutritious Are Fast-Food Meals? *Consumer Reports* (May 1975).

*Hunter, B. T. *The Natural Foods Primer*. New York: Simon and Schuster, 1972.

Index of Nutrition Education Materials. Washington, DC: Nutrition Foundation, 1977.

Journal of Applied Nutrition. International College of Applied Nutrition, La Habra, CA, 1974-76.

*Karelitz, Samuel. *When Your Child Is Ill*. New York: Random House, 1969.

Katz, Marcella. *Vitamins, Food, and Your Health*. Public Affairs Committee, 1971, 1975.

*Kordel, L. *Health Through Nutrition*. New York: MacFadden-Bartell, 1971.

*Linde, Shirley. *The Whole Health Catalog*. New York: Rawson Associates Publishers, 1977.

*Lucas, Richard. *Nature's Medicines*. New York: Prentice-Hall, 1966.

*McGinnis, Terri. *The Well Cat Book*. New York: Random House-Bookworks, 1975.

*———. *The Well Dog Book*. New York: Random House-Bookworks, 1974.

"Marijuana: The Health Questions." *Consumer Reports* 40 (March 1975).

*Martin, Clement G. *Low Blood Sugar: The Hidden Menace of Hypoglycemia*. New York: Arco Publishing Co., 1976.

Martin, Marvin. *Great Vitamin Mystery*. Rosemont, IL: National Dairy Council, 1978.

*Mayer, Jean. *A Diet for Living*. New York: David McKay, 1975.

Mitchell, Helen S. "Recommended Dietary Allowances Up to Date." *Journal of the American Dietetic Association* 64 (February 1974).

National Health Federation Bulletin. November 1973.

National Research Council. *Recommended Dietary Allowances*. 8th ed., revised. Washington, DC: National Academy of Sciences, 1974.

National Research Council. *Toxicants Occurring Naturally in Foods*. 2nd ed. Washington, DC: National Academy of Sciences, 1973.

*Newbold, H. L. *Dr. Newbold's Revolutionary New*

Discovery About Weight Loss. New York: Rawson Associates Publishers, 1977.

———. Mega-Nutrients for Your Nerves. New York: Peter H. Wyden, Publisher, 1973.

*Null, Gary. *The Natural Organic Beauty Book*. New York: Dell, 1972.

*Null, Gary and Steve. *The Complete Book of Nutrition*. New York: Dell, 1972.

**Nutrition Almanac*. New York: McGraw-Hill, 1973.

Nutrition—Applied Personality. La Habra, CA: International College of Applied Nutrition, 1978.

Nutrition Information Resources for the Whole Family. National Nutrition Education Clearing House, 1978.

Nutrition Labeling: How It Can Work for You. National Nutrition Consortium, American Dietetic Association, 1975.

Nutrition Source Book. Rosemont, IL: National Dairy Council, 1978.

"Organic Chemicals in Water: A Major Health Concern." *Consumer Reports* (February 1983):69.

*Passwater, Richard A. *Super Nutrition*. New York: Dial, 1975.

*Pauling, Linus. *Vitamin C and the Common Cold.* New York: Bantam Books, 1971.

*Pearson, Durk, and Shaw, Sandy. *Life Extension*. New York: Warner Books, 1983.

Piltz, Albert. *How Your Body Uses Food*. Rosemont, IL: National Dairy Council, 1960.

*Pommery, Jean. *What to Do till the Veterinarian Comes.* Radnor, PA: Chilton Book Company, 1976.

"Present Knowledge in Nutrition." *Nutrition Reviews*. Nutrition Foundation, Inc., 1976.

*Rodale, J. I. *The Complete Book of Minerals for Health*. 4th ed. Emmaus, PA: Rodale Books, 1976.

*————. *The Encyclopedia of Common Diseases*. Emmaus, PA: Rodale Press, 1976.

*Rosenberg, Harold, and Feldzaman, A. N. *Doctor's Book of Vitamin Therapy: Megavitamins for Health*. New York: Putnam's, 1974.

*Seaman, Barbara and Gideon. *Women and the Crisis in Sex Hormones*. New York: Rawson Associates Publishers, 1977.

*Shute, Wilfrid E., and Taub, Harold J. *Vitamin E for Ailing and Healthy Hearts*. New York: Pyramid Books, 1969.

*Spock, Benjamin. *Baby and Child Care*. New York: Simon and Schuster, 1976.

"Too Much Sugar." *Consumer Reports* 43 (March 1973).

Underwood, Eric J. *Trace Elements in Human and Animal Nutrition*. 4th ed. New York: Academic Press, 1977.

United Nations. Food and Agriculture Organization. *Calorie Requirements,* 1957, 1972.

U.S. Department of Agriculture. *Amino Acid Content of Food* by M. L. Orr and B. K. Watt, 1957; rev. 1968.

U.S. Department of Agriculture. Consumer and Food Economics Institute, Agricultural Research Service. *Composition of Foods: Raw, Processed, Prepared* by Bernice K. Watt and Annabel L. Merrill, 1975.

U.S. Department of Agriculture. *Energy Value of Foods: Basis and Derivation* by Annabel L. Merrill and Bernice K. Watt, 1973.

U.S. Department of Agriculture. *Nutritive Value of American Foods* by Catherine F. Adams, 1975.

U.S. Department of Health, Education and Welfare. *Consumer Health Education: A Directory,* 1975.

U.S. Department of Health, Education and Welfare.

Ten-State Nutrition Survey. Washington, DC: U.S. Government Printing Office, 1968–70.

"The U.S. Food and Drug Administration: On Food and Drugs." *Consumer Reports* 38 (March 1973).

U.S. President's Council on Physical Fitness and Sports. *Exercise and Weight Control* by Robert E. Johnson. Urbana, IL: University of Illinois Press, 1967.

U.S. Senate. Select Committee on Nutrition and Human Needs. *Diet and Killer Diseases with Press Reaction and Additional Information.* Washington, DC: U.S. Government Printing Office, 1977.

U.S. Senate. Select Committee on Nutrition and Human Needs. *National Nutrition Policy: Nutrition and the Consumer II.* Washington, DC: U.S. Government Printing Office, 1974.

"Vitamin-Mineral Safety, Toxicity and Misuse." *Journal of the American Dietetic Association,* 1978.

*Wade, Carlson. *Magic Minerals.* West Nyack, NY: Parker Publishing Co., 1967.

*———. *Miracle Protein.* West Nyack, NY: Parker Publishing Co., 1975.

*———. *Vitamin E: The Rejuvenation Vitamin.* New York: Award Books, 1970.

"Which Cereals Are Most Nutritious?" *Consumer Reports* 40 (February 1975).

Williams, Roger J. *Nutrition Against Disease.* New York: Pitman Publishers, 1971.

*Winter, Ruth. *A Consumer's Dictionary of Food Additives.* New York: Crown, 1973.

*Young, Klein, Beyer. *Recreational Drugs.* New York: Macmillan, 1977.

*Yudkin, John. *Sweet and Dangerous.* New York: Peter H. Wyden, 1972.

Index

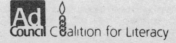